A CHILD'S RECOVERY from AUTISM

Hanna Rotbaum

ISBN: 13: 978-1481289917

CONTENTS

Acknowledgements

First and foremost I thank my friend the editor and artist Linley Eathorne who worked tirelessly with me on this project over the last three years, and without whom the book would never have happened. Her optimism, hard work, editing skills and support kept me going when I might otherwise have faltered. She also made the cover for the book.

I also thank Amy Yasko, Steven Gutstein, and Rachelle Sheely for their extraordinary contribution to advancing the understanding of autism and making my son's recovery possible – and for taking time out of their busy lives to read the book and give feedback. To all the professionals and friends who helped me along the way, I give heartfelt appreciation.

Foreword

After a lifetime of overcoming tough challenges, I used to think that I could do anything if I just tried hard enough. After all, I had overcome the odds and changed my world! Hard work and tenacity had always paid off for me, but having a child with autism was a challenge of an altogether different magnitude. In face of this seemingly insurmountable, baffling, and defeating circumstance, all my previous self-esteem and confidence just drained away. Everything was turned upside down, and it seemed as if I had been thrust into a completely unknown world. I was lost. Things started closing down around me, and a life in prison began. Before I start to tell Jimmy's – and inevitably also my own – story, I need to write about my life before motherhood, as I am convinced that it was my earlier hard life experiences that gave me the strength and determination to help my son overcome autism.

Here is my story:
I was born in East Germany, back when it was a communist country. A wall separated the East from the West. Growing up behind that wall, I felt as if the West might as well have been another planet. It was common knowledge that any attempt to cross the border would be met with deadly force. People simply got shot if they tried to escape. We were prisoners in a grey world. The general atmosphere was full of a muted fear, and caution was the order of the day. We often met our friends in coffee houses but we could not discuss how we really felt about our government. A neighbor, or even one of our

friends, could have been a member of the communist party and quite capable of making the phone call that would have us arrested. Some of my very own friends had been put in prison for political reasons. One of them had painted a West German flag on his bedroom wall; another had made plans to escape. Of course all this had a disheartening and dampening effect on us, but at the same time I was fascinated by the stories of these brave friends who had risked so much, and I too dreamt about a life in freedom.

The prescribed reading in East Germany was the works of the communist theorists Marx and Engels, and though I started out reading such authors, soon I switched to a different kind of literature. My elder brother was friends with a bookstore manager, who passed on to me some almost impossible to find works by authors such as Hermann Hesse, the Nobel Prize winning writer whose novels so brilliantly explore the individual's search for self-knowledge and spirituality. Such books inspired me and opened a window in my mind.

As a young teenager I felt increasingly trapped and depressed about living under such an oppressive totalitarian regime, and not a day went by when I was not thinking about how to escape. My parents refused to join the communist party, since that would have necessitated breaking all ties with our West German relatives. This was understandable, as my father had many close relatives in the West, but the price for not joining the Party was a high one. It meant that my parents had little chance of being promoted in their work lives and that high school education was denied to my siblings and me. One could say our family life was blotted by communism. A great many people joined the communist party for purely practical reasons - simply in order to have access to a slightly better life and more opportunities.

My parents struggled to raise my three brothers and myself on a very small income. My mom was a waitress, and my father was a train conductor. Life was reduced to the basics. There were not a lot of options, since usually the government told you what to think and what to do. My hard-working parents had no choice but to work fulltime in shifts, and my poor mother was working evenings and weekends, leaving us children in childcare from a very early age.

We shared an apartment with an old lady on the third floor. The house was in bad condition, and we didn't even have a bathroom to ourselves. In the often-icy winters, coal was the only available heating source, and it was in very short supply. My parents had to carry the coal up three floors – all the way from the basement – and, sometimes, to keep us from freezing, my father had to scavenge along the train tracks to find the pieces of coal that had fallen off the trains. There was no phone in the apartment, and, like most families, we did not own a car. My parents raised us as best they could. Looking back, I realize how brave and strong my mother was. I don't know how she raised four children in a tiny one-bedroom apartment. I remember all of us sleeping in one room, crawling over each other's beds to get into our own. I clearly recall the endless chores that awaited me after my long school day. Every Friday I waited for hours in line to buy meat for the family. You had to go very early in the morning to have any chance of getting meat. When there were vegetables at the market, hundreds of people would stand for hours in line just to buy a few tomatoes.

As a teenager I became difficult and rebellious and too much for my poor parents to handle. Of course most teenagers have a rebellious period. I felt my individuality was being ignored. I was not being "seen" for who I was, and I was flailing against the myriad of restrictions that made up my life. It got so bad that my parents decided I would have to leave home when I turned eighteen.

The year that followed was very bleak. Unable to find a place to live, I was reduced to sleeping on the floor in various friends' apartments. I felt depressed and isolated, with no clear way ahead for myself in East Germany. What future could there be for me without a good education and always being discriminated against for not being a communist! After much anguish I decided to somehow find a way to escape. The year was 1989. The only possibility was to get to West Germany via Poland, the Czech Republic, Hungary and Austria. Escaping seemed more possible than before, since the Hungarian government had already opened the border to Austria. From there it would be just a matter of crossing the border to West Germany. Getting any exit visa was extremely tough, but fortunately I managed to get an invitation to visit from a friend in Hungary. This was my key to freedom. I applied for the visa and felt strangely confident that this would indeed work out.

About a month later with the miracle of my Hungarian visa in my pocket, I set off full of wild excitement and determination. I would take my future in my hands and start a completely new and better life. I gave little thought to the consequences of failure and turned the fear dancing around my heart into iron resolve. In each country armed soldiers searched me for any clues that might indicate an intention to escape. For this reason I carried very little with me. If the soldiers had found anything suspicious, I would have been arrested and incarcerated. Somehow my inner agitation seemed not to communicate itself to the soldiers who, though extraordinarily thorough in their questioning and searches, let me pass at every checkpoint.

After four nerve wracking days of traveling on slow trains and staying in cheap hotels, I finally found myself safe in the free world. I looked around me in amazement and delight. All those pretty little well-kept Austrian villages brought home to me that I was now indeed in another place. I could breathe out at last! From there I continued to the gloriously beautiful Bavaria, West Germany. I faced my new life almost like a newborn child. There I stood with just two shirts, two pairs of pants and no money at all!

West Germany was welcoming. I was granted refugee status, given a place to stay, and, fortunately, soon found a job as a waitress in a

Bavarian village. Being in a free country, I could finally begin my high school studies – at twenty-six years of age! Getting my high school diploma was not exactly easy. I was working full time as a waitress, and in the evening I took high school classes. Being unable to work the late shift, however, I was soon fired from the restaurant. Needing to support myself, I then had to take any job I could get and eventually started working at a chicken farm, sorting eggs at a conveyer belt all day or stuffing live chickens in tiny cages. The work conditions were dreadful. I worked six days a week, laboring all day in dust and dirt without water or food.

Sometimes I had to go back at night to take the chickens out of the cages for slaughtering. I felt terrible about this, and I wished I could have rescued every single chicken. But since I needed the money, I just had to grit my teeth and keep on going. It was tough finding enough time to study so I used to take my history book to the farm, reading furtively while stuffing empty egg boxes into the conveyer belt. I had to be very careful, as I couldn't afford to lose my job. This all paid off in the end, and at the ripe old age of twenty-nine I finally received my high school diploma with special merit. Doors now opened up before me. A dream had really come true.

With my new, hard-earned high school diploma I enrolled in a university studying for a Masters in Psychology. This was the best time of my life. There was nothing to be afraid of any more. Every morning I woke up incredibly happy and excited to go off to the library to read whatever I wanted. My West German student friends were rather surprised that I missed all the parties, and they could not understand how anybody could possibly spend all day in the library. It felt so good to be free. Soon I even got accepted as an exchange student to go to America – the land of endless possibilities in my dreams. As I joyously set off for studies at the University of Colorado, Boulder, part of me could not believe the extraordinary turn of events. Could this really be me?

When I arrived in Boulder, it was total English immersion for me, as English was never taught in East Germany. Luckily, soon after my arrival there, I met my future husband, who helped me master this completely new language. Being in love is certainly the best way to learn a new language! Marrying an American would change my whole life once more. America was a very foreign and exciting place to me, and after all the years of cultural deprivation I threw myself into catching up by enthusiastically exploring art museums, going to theater performances and immersing myself in music of all kinds. We reveled in the easy sociability of student life in the West. After all the hard experiences of my early life, I felt like a new and strong person ready to meet whatever would come. But as it turned out, nothing had prepared me for the challenge of having an autistic child.

When my son was diagnosed with autism, I wish I had known then what I have written about in this book. I invite all involved parents, relatives and teachers to read my son's story. It is not only about Jimmy's recovery, it also describes the tremendous stresses autism can inflict upon an affected family. It tells of my own limitations and the strength granted me through the love of my child, to carry us through to where we are today. I have attempted to distill what I learned through years of trial and error and hard experience, into useful tips and pointers to smooth the way for people still struggling with all the challenges autism brings. I hope this book will make a difference.

Chapter One

THE PRELUDE

Expectations of Motherhood

I was completely unprepared for the roller-coaster life with my autistic son. How could anybody be adequately prepared to face such a thing? But of course it had to be faced and I did face it, and there has even been a good outcome. I still ask myself how on earth I found the wherewithal to cope with it all.

A Hard East German Childhood

When I look back now at my hard childhood in East Germany I can see that the strength that has carried me through must have come at least partly from surviving my difficult childhood. And when I look back at that childhood, it seems almost improbable that I should be where I am today: living in a foreign country with a good standard of living, married, and with my own child. Having an autistic child has meant I have come through testing times again. Though of course I would never wish such a thing on anyone, it has matured me and changed my outlook on life profoundly.

Given that I grew up thinking of motherhood as a burdensome, imprisoning, and grim undertaking, it is surprising that I ever embraced having a family of my own. I am amazed at the chasms that have been bridged. Certainly getting married was not on my agenda at all, and as a young woman, I couldn't think why anyone would get married and have children.

This extreme position stems from life in the so-called German Democratic Republic or DDR as it was mostly called. I say "so-called," as there was nothing remotely democratic about it. Living under this system was no walk in the park, and my parents' already difficult lives were made so much harder by having to raise four children on very little money. To make our lives manageable they instituted a rigid discipline in our household. To escape the crushing effect of this, I spent whatever small amount of spare time I had at the riding school on the edge of our town: cleaning out stalls or watching other people ride. I was mad about horses, and I dreamed of one day having my own horse and having a completely different life. Sometimes I even got to ride the horses, and then I was in heaven.

When I came home dirty and smelling of stables, my mother was not pleased, to put it mildly. In those pre-washing-machine days, all clothes had to be washed by hand and then hung out to dry on the clothesline. I still remember the smell of the cotton clothes my mother boiled in a big pot. Often, I lost my shoes playing in the mud or ripped my clothes climbing horse fences. Back in East Germany, clothes and shoes were not easily replaced, and good shoes were rare.

Other children there seemed to have much more freedom than I did, and I rebelled against this strict and restrictive environment in any way I could. It seemed clear to me that I was simply a burden to the family, and tensions were high. Almost inevitably, I ended up leaving home as soon as I could.

"Freedom" Leads Nowhere

The rush of pleasure at being finally "free" was short lived as the realities of so-called independent living soon hit me hard. It was not easy to find an apartment in East Germany and usually people had to put their names on a waiting list. It could take up to ten years or longer to get approved for an apartment. There I was supposedly free, but I had no place to go.

For months I moved around from one friend's home to another's, until one night in the depths of a cold winter, I found myself out on the streets alone with only a suitcase. Freezing and desperate, I eventually found refuge in a rundown bed and breakfast. It was horrible and uncomfortable, but at least I had somewhere to go after work. This reprieve from homelessness was short lived, however, as the owner threw me out after two weeks for the high crime of washing laundry in the sink! Laundromats did not exist in East Germany. I was saved from staying in the streets by the compassion of a colleague who took me in for over a year until I finally got my own apartment. This was a very low period of my life, and I still shudder to think of what might have happened if this big-hearted colleague had not come to my rescue.

Cutting Off My Parents

After my escape to West Germany, my anger and resentment towards my parents grew. I blamed them for not helping me with my education, and eventually I refused to have any contact with them. For ten whole years, I cut them out of my life. I didn't see them, I didn't write them, and I never called them.

Looking back on it all now, I realize that I was very immature. After the wall came down, my poor parents were still struggling in East Germany. After the reunification with the West, the unemployment rate in the East skyrocketed, and my parents were not sure if they would be able to keep their jobs and support themselves. Back then I paid very little attention to their predicament. Cutting them off was easier for me at that time, as I was so focused on my new way forward.

The Shift Towards Settling Down

I was already in my thirties doing graduate studies in West Germany when my sour view of family life changed. I witnessed my friends getting married and having children, and as I watched them show off their beautiful babies I was struck by how happy they were. I began looking forward to visiting them and playing with their children. For the first time I realized that children could be a true joy – and not just work and worry to their parents.

In graduate school I became friends with a fellow student who was dreaming about finding the right partner and having her own family. Although back then I was not in the least interested in settling down, I became fascinated by the optimistic way she saw the world, and this caused my perspectives to shift. The prospect of a settled relationship leading to marriage started to look appealing for the very first time.

At that time, I thought I knew what kind of person I was looking for – someone attractive, highly intelligent and responsible with a stable job. I was lucky to be at a big university where there were plenty of interesting young men and very soon I found a wonderful boyfriend who shared my life goals. It was incredibly exciting. My life was just starting, and I had never felt better.

Soon, I was accepted as an exchange student in the United States. I had always been fascinated by America, which to me symbolized freedom and independence. Though it would be difficult to leave my boyfriend behind, I had to take advantage of this once in a lifetime opportunity. I could not wait to arrive in America. Little did I know what challenges life there would bring me.

Once in America, I realized that actually living in a foreign country was not at all the same thing as taking a vacation there. I struggled quite a lot with the completely unfamiliar culture, but in time with help from my new American friends, I settled in.

Among the group of students I moved around with there
was an engineering student with whom I soon became close. This presented a problem as I was in love with my boyfriend back in Germany, wasn't I? Complications notwithstanding, my American boyfriend and I found ourselves falling very much in love, and in time marriage followed. We decided our future life would be in America.

Marriage and a New Life in California

A small group of friends watched us take our vows in northern California, and a few days later we went off for our honeymoon. This was everything a honeymoon should be. A romantic bed and breakfast place right on the ocean and perfect weather. Luck smiled on us when we ended up in the most expensive room with a huge jacuzzi. We could never have afforded this, but it came our way as an apology for the manager having forgotten about our reservation. Golden days followed as we rode horses on the beach and watched the sea lions and were simply happy. I am so glad we had this special time together, because there were many years to follow when my husband and I would spend no time together alone at all. I still wish we could have stayed there longer.

Due to having relatives in so many distant places, we had two more wedding receptions, one in France and one in Colorado. This was a magical time and all the more precious because of what was to come after our son was born. Everything was so perfect that I naively imagined that life would always be that happy.

We had rented a little house in Berkeley near San Francisco. Our social life there was very active, and we were constantly partying. However it didn't take long for this kind of lifestyle to pall, and I started feeling distance towards the friends of that time who were mostly artists or musicians in their twenties or early thirties, all trying to find themselves in some way. I, on the other hand, was tired of moving around and was feeling the need for more stability. By that time I had traveled widely in Europe and North America and had moved house far too many times. Now that I was married, life needed to be different. I was so ready to take care of another human being. Yes, I wanted a baby. I was 35 years old.

Preparation for Becoming a Mother

As a first step to motherhood I joined a mother's book club to educate myself about pregnancy. I learned about eating the healthiest foods and avoiding alcohol. Although I wasn't even pregnant yet, I found out everything I could about birthing classes and breastfeeding support groups. I often visited 4th Street in Berkeley, where I loved sitting in a café watching mothers and fathers pushing their beautiful babies in their carriages. They looked so happy. I pictured myself being one of them. It never crossed my mind that motherhood could be anything other than this.

When we got a positive pregnancy test result, we felt very lucky. I felt reassured that I had done everything right and that everything would go according to plan. I was aware that the beginning of the pregnancy could be critical, because I had known people who had lost their baby within the first three months. After regular check-ups I had an ultrasound examination that showed images of the baby, amniotic sac, placenta, and ovaries. It can detect major anatomical abnormalities or birth defects. My doctor reassured me my baby was healthy and I believed him. I was watching my body for anything that was out of the ordinary. Morning sickness took hold but that, unfortunately, was quite normal, and soon my pregnancy started to show.

In my reading I paid special attention to the risks of pregnancy. I learned that women in my age group have a higher chance of having a baby with Downs Syndrome. Miscarriage, pregnancy complications and cesarean births also increase with age. I found out about amniocentesis, a diagnostic test that allows a woman either to terminate a pregnancy or help prepare her for the special needs her baby might have. The books said little about other complications and nowhere did I see a mention of autism. When I was fifteen weeks pregnant, my doctor offered an amniocentesis test and I decided to go ahead with it, as it could provide a lot of information. Later I realized that such a test has a 0.5 percent chance of causing a miscarriage. Luckily, the results showed our baby was well and free of birth defects.

Attachment Parenting

Now I just needed to find the perfect parenting approach. This shouldn't be hard for me, given the time I had spent studying child development at college. I had already learnt about different parenting styles, and I think as a reaction to my childhood I wanted to raise my child in a child-centered approach. I loved the book by William Sears and Martha Sears espousing a parenting style called "attachment parenting." This highly responsive, attentive style of caring for a child promotes physical and emotional closeness between parent and child. I loved the idea of carrying my baby in a sling and breastfeeding on demand.

La Leche League

Having read about complications with breast-feeding, I decided to go to La Leche League meetings. La Leche League was founded in 1956 by five women from Illinois and has since expanded into more than 63 countries. It is a charitable organization offering free practical information and moral support to mothers through monthly meetings, e-mails, phone calls, and websites. I learned that breastfed babies had a lower risk of developing respiratory illnesses, ear infections, stomach viruses and meningitis. Exclusive breastfeeding for at least six months provided the most protection. Its proponents held that it could even reduce the risk of childhood cancer, type one and type two diabetes, high cholesterol and inflammatory bowel disease in later life. Apparently it could also lower the risk of obesity and boost a child's intelligence. I was convinced I would be a great mother with the knowledge I was gaining and with all the support groups I attended.

Mending Broken Fences and Revisiting My Past

Starting a family opened a door for me to reconnect with my parents. I certainly wanted my child to have a relationship with its grandparents and I had by this time gotten beyond blaming them for my past unhappiness and failures. Before getting married I had summoned up courage and written to invite my parents to my wedding. This was doubtless quite a shock for them after ten years of silence, and they were not ready to accept the invitation. More time was needed for them to get used to their "new" daughter.

Gradually over many phone conversations we began to rebuild a relationship and became at ease with one another. This reconciliation was cemented when we accepted their invitation to visit them in Germany. They welcomed us there in such a heart-felt way that my husband felt at home immediately. Soon it was clear to me that my ten-year absence was forgiven. They looked at their new son-in-law with pride in their eyes, and I sensed they were very happy. My parents were plainly relieved that their wayward daughter had come to the realization of the value of family and were also delighted that I was going to have a child.

Being back in Germany, pregnant, and getting ready to be a mother made me think about my biological mother. Sadly, I don't remember her at all, as she died when I was just one-and-a-half years old. That was around 1968. It was said she died from eating poisonous mushrooms she had collected with some friends. However her death was documented as "unnatural" or as being from "external causes." None of the other people with her had died or even gotten sick.

Strangely, although police procedure back then required such a death to be investigated, the East German police never investigated. It was generally known that poisoning was a common method used by the Stasi for getting rid of "anti-communists." The background to my mother's untimely death remains murky. She did have contacts to West German friends and had lived for some time in West Germany, but perhaps there was more to it than that? Perhaps, one day this will be cleared up.

Moving to Boston and the Birth of Our Healthy Baby

Just one month before I gave birth we moved from San Francisco to Boston, as my husband had a new post-doctoral position in a lab at Harvard. Everything seemed rosy and full of promise. I had been a methadone counselor and was working towards a Marriage and Family Therapy license in San Francisco. I was confident that I would be working again six months after the birth.

My son came into this world on a beautiful sunny day in September.

Apparently, there was nothing extraordinary about the birth. Like most new mothers I had little understanding of alternatives to drugs during the birth. When the doctors gave me Pitocin to induce labor, I had no idea of the possible side effects, which included fetal distress and increased need for a Cesarean section birth and an epidural – as occurred in my case. Epidural anesthesia is a widely used method of pain relief during labor, and over half the women in the US choose to have an epidural. It is generally considered safe, but several possible side effects are increased risk of urinary tract infection, headaches, itching, drop in blood pressure, and fever. In rare cases, allergic shock, convulsions, respiratory paralysis, cardiac arrest and maternal death have occurred. Overall the birthing process did seem to me to be more of a medical procedure than a natural event. The doctors and nurses told me what to do, and I was a compliant patient.

Years later, after watching a documentary about natural childbirth, I wished I had been given the option of giving birth in a non-invasive and un-medicated way. I wish I had questioned modern ways of giving birth and understood more about how women have historically given birth naturally, without being overpowered by medical professionals.

When I saw my son for the first time, I thought he had the cutest little face. He looked right at me. A miracle had happened. A whole train of medical professionals measured and tested him with great thoroughness. Once again we were reassured that we had a healthy baby. My husband and I couldn't have been happier.

Post Partum Blues

- Up to eighty percent of mothers feel moody, weepy and anxious during the first two weeks after giving birth.
- Postpartum depression can occur any time in the first six months and usually lasts longer than two weeks.
- Mothers often feel upset, alone, afraid, or even sometimes unloving toward the baby. In addition there are often deep feelings of guilt about having these feelings.

The day I had to leave the hospital I had a sudden failure of confidence. Did I just have the "baby blues" or was it the beginning of postpartum depression? My happiness turned into anxiety. I was terrified. I refused to leave the hospital, and I insisted there was no way I would be able to take care of such a helpless human being. The nurses kept reassuring me that it was quite normal to feel scared, and that a lot of new mothers have those feelings. Later at home, when I gently put the baby on our bed and wrapped him into a blanket, I found myself smiling broadly. He looked just like a burrito with only his little face sticking out.

Luckily my sister-in-law arrived to help with cooking and taking care of Jimmy. This support made all the difference and her calmness and confidence helped me get over my anxiety. My husband seemed very calm and confident as well. He became an expert in changing diapers and wrapping Jimmy in blankets. At night we took turns rocking him back to sleep after he woke up.

My husband had taken time off work but would have return to work soon. My sister-in-law needed to go back to France as well, and then I would be alone with the baby. That day arrived too soon, but slowly Jimmy and I found our own routine, and finally I started to feel more confident. Breastfeeding stayed painful for a while, but with the help of breastfeeding support meetings I managed to continue doing it.

I Love My Baby

Jimmy seemed easy to take care of: he barely cried and was a happy baby. By the age of two months he started sleeping through the night, gaining weight and growing. His weight was about average, and there was no cause for any concern. I was so proud of myself. Everything was going so well. Soon I joined a mothers' group in the hospital where I had given birth. Back then I was just the same as the other mothers. I was in love with my beautiful baby, and everybody in my new mothers' group commented on Jimmy, how beautiful he was and how well he was developing. It felt so good to be part of the joy of motherhood. I loved discussing baby clothes, breast-feeding and developmental milestones with the other mothers.

After the group we went out for lunch holding our babies on our laps or letting them sleep peacefully in their strollers. We talked and painted pictures of our children's future. Since Jimmy slept most of the time in the afternoon, I could easily take him to the movies. I was so happy to have so much company, and the days went by too quickly.

I became very close friends with one mother who later would turn out to be my lifesaver. I instantly liked Penny and loved listening to what she had to say. Often she would bring her first son who was a high-spirited toddler at this time. She talked to me about the challenges she had with him during babyhood, about how he had cried incessantly and had other challenging behaviors and sensory issues. She told me her son cried so much and so loudly that she had to wear headphones to be with him. I had never heard anything like it. Somehow I was drawn to her and after a while we started meeting at the local café, drinking warm tea in that cold Boston winter. I imagined our boys happily playing together once they were older.

Of course when you have a baby you have to take it for regular check ups. I did not really know what to look for in a pediatrician even though I had researched countless sites on the Internet and had read parenting journals.

How to Find a Good Pediatrician

Articles on this subject usually emphasize that one should look for a pediatrician with

- medical training at reputable institutions
- extensive experience
- short waiting time.

With my experience, I would add some other important qualities to look for.

For example:

- ❖ willing to listen to the parent, as opposed to simply giving orders
- ❖ trained thoroughly in infant nutrition, developmental abnormalities, and social development
- ❖ does not give antibiotics every time the child has a runny nose
- ❖ willing to explore natural therapeutic alternatives
- ❖ respectful of my parenting approach

My pediatrician usually saw my son for five minutes and asked me about eating and sleeping habits. He was concerned mostly about my son's height and weight and didn't ask many questions about his social development. He always reassured me that our son was doing very well, and as he told me there was nothing at all to worry about, I was content. I had a healthy beautiful son and a loving supportive family. What could possibly go wrong?

Chapter 2

RECOGNIZING AUTISM

Jimmy started to change at the age of three months, but as he was my first child and I had no idea what normal child development looked like, it didn't register that anything could be seriously wrong. New mothers are often so overloaded just coping with the daily needs of the baby that it wouldn't even enter their minds that there could be a developmental problem. On top of feeling overloaded and deprived of sleep, first-time mothers experience hormonal changes often leaving them feeling anxious and low. Thus it is not at all surprising that autism symptoms remain unnoticed by parents in the early stages. Nonetheless, as scientists now believe signs of autism can often be detected within the first twelve months, pediatricians should ideally be watchful of possible developmental red flags in early infancy. Intervention can be beneficial at any age, though it seems that the earlier the intervention, the better the outcome.

Achieving an early diagnosis would be made easier if new parents knew what typical development looks like. Of course, there is considerable variation in early milestones and most people know stories of the child who uttered no word for the first three years and then brought forth entire sentences. Generally though, babies should be babbling by one year and using words such as "ook" for "book" or "uice" for "juice" by about fifteen months. By the end of their first year infants are naturally interested in each other, and they imitate clapping or waving good-bye. They should be orienting towards something you are pointing to, or they point to get your attention.

Some professionals indicate that parents should watch out for two important early ways of communicating. These are referencing and experience sharing. From a very early age typical children keep track of their parents' whereabouts. They observe their parents' reactions in uncertain situations and adjust their behavior based on their parents' reactions. For example, they bring a toy to the caregiver to see what their reaction is. Is this a safe toy? Is it important? The adult becomes the reference point for the child. In experience sharing, the infant communicates enjoyment by smiling and gazing at the parents face when, for example, they change simple games and songs. In nursery songs and games such as Peekaboo, these interactions happen naturally between parents and babies.

Parents might be able to detect impaired reference and experience sharing skills even in the first year of life. Looking back now I realize that in his first year Jimmy did definitely show symptoms of early autism. He rarely pointed or showed me toys to see what I thought of them. He was unable to find me even when I was right next to him. He did not like it when I added new elements in a game, and even small changes in routines would upset him terribly. His gestures and understanding of gestures were very limited. He communicated only if he wanted something such as his bear or food. When you are a new mother it is not always easy to clearly see these things.

Although many autistic children do manifest early symptoms, today most children are not diagnosed until two or three years of age, because it is thought that a later diagnosis would be more accurate. Also many pediatricians believe a later diagnosis would avoid unnecessary and costly intervention. However, many parents would prefer an early diagnosis so they could start treating their children as soon as possible and indeed getting started sooner might well cost less in the long run.

One common obstacle in diagnosing autism is that it is a spectrum disorder. Although autistic children have a variety of symptoms in common, they differ greatly in personality, mood and intelligence, as well as in the severity of their symptoms. They may also have other conditions such as sensory integration dysfunction, gastrointestinal sensitivities and various speech deficits. These conditions could mask autism and complicate an early diagnosis.

In our case, when Jimmy was resistant to play, the occupational therapist thought this was just because he was overly sensitive to touch. She overlooked completely the high anxiety he showed when she made any changes in the games. For example, any change in the hand holding game "Ring around a Rosie" distressed him so much that he would scream and run away. This symptom could easily have been an early sign of autism

Sensory Dysfunction

Dr. A. Jean Ayres developed the sensory integration theory to explain the relationship between behavior and brain function. Supporters of this theory believe that dysfunction results from the brain's inability to integrate, process, and respond to sensory information – such as from smell, sight, taste, sound, temperature, pain and movements. Children can either over- or under-react to stimulation. For example, a toddler who has difficulty integrating tactile (touch) input may avoid unpleasant touch experiences such as getting his hands messy with paint, sand, or glue, while another child may crave such touch input and actively seek it out. Other symptoms of this dysfunction include over- or under-sensitivity to movement, sights, or sounds, as well as difficulties in regulation of emotions and social development.

Jimmy started showing a variety of symptoms of this dysfunction from three months of age. He changed from being happy and content to being very unhappy and constantly screaming. Anything could set him off: a sudden movement, a door closed too loudly, a toy falling out of his hand, being exposed to bright sunlight, a runny nose, or being put down for a second.

Changing and dressing Jimmy became a nightmare, because he could not tolerate the feel of clothes on his body. It was so sad that he couldn't wear all the new outfits my family had sent from Germany. I could only imagine how cute he would have looked in them. As it was, simply getting him into or out of any clothing could make him scream for over an hour. In addition, his being so overly sensitive to certain noises limited severely what we could do as a family. Sneezes or clapping would completely terrify him, and any kind of noise at all would be enough to wake him.

It wasn't until two years later that Jimmy got occupational therapy to help him with his sensory integration. However many of the therapy techniques he received at that time could have been applied as early as three months, especially the Wilbarger protocol treatment regime designed to reduce sensory defensiveness. This treatment includes brushing the child with a special brush and this I could easily have done in those early days. It could have greatly reduced his aversion to touch and might have improved his sleeping patterns. And, of course, it would have saved us all a great deal of grief as well.

Extreme Sleep Issues

When Jimmy reached three months of age, his sleeping habits also began to change, until it became so extreme that he was waking up about every ten minutes. As no naps seemed to last longer than five minutes I became so dangerously sleep deprived that I was very close to the end of my tether. I felt uncomprehending as I held this tiny body so clearly deeply exhausted. How could such exhaustion not bring about sleep! Sometimes before dawn I would put him in the stroller and go out walking in the hope it might calm him down.

In desperation I started seeing the pediatrician twice a week but all he came up with was that I was just a new mother and too nervous around the baby. Those severe sleeping issues should have been a red flag and cause for a closer investigation of developmental issues, but he insisted that I was the problem. This was very hard to bear. I read every book about sleep problems on the market and most of them believed comforting the crying baby in the crib reinforces staying awake. Instead, the baby should be left crying for short periods of time to give it a chance to fall asleep. There is so much advice on this question and much of it conflicting.

In some books they recommended the parent stay in the room while others advised the parent to leave. A few experts advocated co-sleeping, meaning the baby sleeps with the parents. We had already practiced co-sleeping but without success, so we decided to give Jimmy some time to fall asleep on his own. I hated leaving him in his crib all alone, but I just had to get some sleep in order to function. Jimmy did manage to sleep longer periods of time with this method but it took him years before he could sleep through the night.

The Destructive Effect Upon the Family

Living with a screaming, non-sleeping child can have a very destructive effect on a family. I had to carry Jimmy around all the time, walking very carefully to avoid sudden movements. With the baby crying over my shoulder, it took me an hour to make a sandwich and two hours to eat it. I was perpetually walking on eggshells trying to avoid making a wrong move.

Living like this became pure hell and as the months dragged on with no change I gradually started going downhill physically and mentally. I got a breast infection and felt so weak that I could barely function. I think I was perilously close to a nervous breakdown. I was dead tired and in so much pain but had to continue breast-feeding night and day as he refused any other food. How could it be so hard to have a baby? How could my mom ever have managed to take care of all four of us? What was I doing wrong, I kept asking myself over and over again. "Just move on," "snap out of it," I heard over and over from family members and friends.

By the time Jimmy turned eleven months, my patience had all but run out, and the stress on our marriage was almost unbearable. In a wave of complete despair, I admitted myself to psychiatric emergency care. The staff were mostly concerned about whether I had any impulses to hurt my baby. I did not. They offered some counseling, but they could not really help me with Jimmy's challenges. They encouraged me to take some time off from the baby, and soon I took this advice and started feeling less guilty about leaving Jimmy with my husband even though I knew it would be hard on him with the baby screaming the whole time I was gone.

Avoiding Peers

When one-year-old children are playing next to each other, they usually do similar activities. They enjoy being near one another, watching and imitating each other. Before age one, Jimmy began developing extreme anxiety towards other children. He started screaming if anyone even came near him. I soon realized there was no point in taking him to baby groups at all.

In spite of this and all my best instincts, I found myself soon joining with a group of local German-speaking mothers and babies, so that Jimmy could learn to interact in German. It had always been one of my greatest wishes to have our son grow up bi-lingual. The plan was to meet every week at different houses. For some reason we ended up most of the time at my place. I used to clean up the house the night before a meeting when Jimmy was asleep. I would prepare snacks, drinks and loads of toys for the babies. When they all arrived, Jimmy would be content usually for only about ten minutes, and then he would start crying loudly – especially when the other toddlers came closer. He just could not be near the other children.

Not wanting to spoil the atmosphere, I told people to make themselves at home, and then I would grab Jimmy and take him for a walk or to the park to calm down. On returning after an hour or longer, usually everybody had left and my house looked as if a tornado had just hit it. So after Jimmy was in bed, I would clean up the house and just cry.

Honestly, I have no idea why I kept on with this over the next months. Perhaps, I was still in a certain amount of denial and still hoped that he would get used to the other children and start enjoying the playgroup. It was equally disastrous at other people's houses. I would be forced to excuse myself and leave after a short time.

Far from improving with time, it seemed to actually get even worse. The other mothers seemed so relaxed with their babies crawling around the room happily exploring all the great toys. They chatted away together leaving me feeling excluded and different. Clearly I was not one of them.

Lack of peer play is one of the symptoms of autism. Children with autism may perceive other children as being too unpredictable, and this can be very overwhelming for them.

Most one year olds will engage in imitative play. They try to act like their parents, using plastic cell phones, pretend to shop and dress up and wear costumes. They pretend to cook and take out your pots and pans. They love to play with plastic plates and foods. It was clear that Jimmy was on a different developmental path than typical children. I bought him lots of toy cars, plastic food items and little play figures, hoping this would encourage him to play.

However, he never engaged in imaginary play or any other meaningful play. Instead, he liked to open and close doors for long periods of time or he would roll a truck back and forth in the same motion. He lined his toys up instead of playing with them. I didn't really know at the time that this was not normal, but of course if I had been aware that this behavior could have indicated autism, I would have started therapy right then.

I think I survived this painful and dreadful time, because of my neighborhood friend Penny. She was there for me whenever I needed her. It was so reassuring to have one person I could count on. She understood my situation and never blamed me. I visited her whenever I got a chance. She would light a comforting fire in the fireplace, make some tea, and we would have some chocolate. I managed to stay only a short time, but with her I had my only moments of relaxation. Somehow, Jimmy could handle being with Penny better than with any other person, but as soon as anybody else was nearby I would have to leave.

Sometimes we talked about her older son and how he had gotten early intervention. She told me about the occupational therapist who had come every week to spend an hour with her son. It was extraordinary that the very same therapist would come to my house two years later. If only I had made the connection then, but at that time, I was still stuck in hoping that one day Jimmy would just wake up and the nightmare would be over.

Trying to Do Normal Things Just Didn't Work

It was a sad fact that at that time that I never felt as if my family understood me at all! All the criticism left me feeling guilty about my ability as a mother and unworthy in general. Just before Christmas my sister-in-law invited us to her friend's house in upstate New York. This was a terrifying prospect since any car journey always provoked hysterical screaming from the baby. Being stuck with him screaming in a small space was an absolute nightmare. My husband insisted that we go, since we had to have some kind of a real life and not just stay at home all the time because of Jimmy.

However, just as I expected, the car ride ended up with Jimmy screaming and my husband and I fighting. We all were very tense when we entered that picture-perfect house, beautifully decorated for Christmas. I hated being there, because I was afraid everybody would see how incompetent I was as a mother.

At the beginning everybody was very nice and tried to help out with the baby, but unfortunately this didn't improve things, as Jimmy's crying intensified when people came near him. I ended up holding the screaming baby as much as I could while everybody else enjoyed celebrating Christmas.

Even during the night there was no respite, and with the heat being turned off at that time, I would find myself in an overcoat walking him back and forth in the kitchen. I was cold, sad and miserable, and everybody knew it. My husband got mad at me for not being able to have a good time. After all, it was Christmas, and people were supposed to be happy! Just thinking about this trip still makes me feel angry and embarrassed. After three days I dug the car out of the snow and insisted on leaving. At this point I didn't care what anybody else was thinking about me, and we set off for home under a big unhappy grey cloud.

Another memorable Christmas was to follow, when my mother-in-law came to visit for three weeks. I had actually looked forward to seeing her and getting some support, as we always had gotten along so well. However this didn't work out well, as my mother-in-law was completely unused to being with a little unhappy bundle crying all the time. Things were tense from the beginning and further deteriorated when she tried to feed Jimmy vegetables. He screamed when she attempted to hold him or even be near him. Patiently she tried to engage him in any kind of play, but Jimmy was interested only in opening and closing doors or watching the water running down the sink.

Once she suggested that what Jimmy really needed was to be out in the countryside in calming green nature. So we duly set off. Understandably, she found the screaming infant so distracting that she ran through a red light. I was afraid I would make her more nervous by mentioning it, so, as the situation was quite bad enough already, I bit my tongue. She told me how happy her kids had been when they were exposed to nature, and how she hoped that once we arrived Jimmy would calm down.

Unfortunately, even the peaceful countryside proved to be too much for Jimmy, and he just cried and fussed the whole time. Completely stressed out, we drove home in near silence. Things became increasingly tense as time went on. On top of all this, she felt hurt that I spent every second with the baby and very little time with her son, my husband. It didn't help that she had to sleep on the living room couch where there was no way to escape the noise. The situation became steadily more impossible, and after two weeks I lost control and told her she would have to find another place to stay. After that we stopped talking to each other for a long time.

I felt wretched about losing contact with this woman whom I liked and admired so much. Things seemed to be falling apart around me. I was a stranger amongst my friends, and I had stopped talking to my family. It never really registered at the time that my son was already developmentally very different from my friends' children.

It never occurred to me that my son, who was not even one year old, showed symptoms of autism. Had I known this, I might have been able to save my son from slipping further into autism, and maybe I could have saved the friendships and relationships with family members. Most parents don't realize that early developmental differences in their child could indicate autism.

If a child shows any developmental delay or misses important developmental milestones, I think pediatricians should alert the parents. It is the parents who are always with their children and can keep a closer eye out for red flags. They should be active partners in the process of finding out if a diagnosis is appropriate. Above all, parents need to be aware what typical development looks like.

Summary of Possible Early Symptoms of Autism

- lack of interest in interaction with peers or parents
- exaggerated and frequent, inconsolable crying
- inability to tolerate even small changes in routine
- extreme sleeping problems
- extreme sensory sensitivity
- language delay
- extreme eating problems
- lack of referencing ability
- missing several of the normal developmental milestones

Each autistic child may very well have a slightly different set of symptoms. The presence of one or more of these symptoms does not necessarily mean the child has autism, but having several could possibly be a red flag. If all or most of the above mentioned are present, then it would be a good idea to take your child to a specialist for investigation.

Trust Your Instincts

I wish I had been strong enough to go against other people's advice. They would usually tell me that Jimmy was the way he was, because I was being overprotective, or they told that all babies cry and that I shouldn't worry. Now after many years I have become very strong and I always trust my instincts. I do listen to what other people have to say, but I know for sure that as Jimmy's mom I really do know best.

Chapter Three

DIAGNOSIS and EARLY INTERVENTION

How Do You Get an Autism Diagnosis?

Autism is a medical condition and usually parents have to see a pediatric neurologist or psychiatrist (MD) for a proper diagnosis of their child. A psychologist (PsyD or PhD), a clinical social worker (MSW or LCSW or LMSW) or a licensed professional counselor (LPC) can also give a diagnosis. However, gaining access to these professionals is by no means easy, as they often have very long waiting lists.

Given that early treatment results in a better outcome, this inaccessibility can be enormously frustrating. Even if the parents do manage to see a professional, they may disagree with the evaluation and may want to get a second or third opinion.

As mentioned in a previous chapter, if parents feel they are not getting appropriate answers, they have to trust their own instincts. They are the ones who see the child on a daily basis, while professionals only see the child briefly. If parents are unable to get a diagnosis, they are likely to have more difficulties finding access to certain treatments but they should persevere, as there are many available therapies. The main obstacle is financial as, generally, no funding for treatment is available without a formal medical diagnosis.

Pediatricians may not be qualified to make an autism diagnosis, as usually they lack specific training. If parents are concerned about their child's lack of typical development, they should schedule a longer visit with their pediatrician and press for a referral to a specialist.

If the pediatrician isn't supportive, this would be time to look elsewhere – preferably for a developmental pediatrician. If your child is under the age of three, and you are unsuccessful in getting any help from professionals, it would be best to call the early intervention program in your town.

As I had no professional support in finding out how to help my son, I read any book I could lay my hands on about developmental disabilities in children. I had the feeling that the answers to all my questions were written down somewhere. I searched through so many stories about mothers struggling just as I was, in the hope I would find a case similar to my own. I read and I read, and then one day just before Jimmy's second birthday, I finally found him!

Here was an entire book about this one boy who was diagnosed with autism and it was as if I was reading about my own son. I was dying and reborn at the same time. If Jimmy did have autism, it would be a lifelong incurable condition. This felt terrible, but it would take away the crushing weight about it being all my fault.

The story was not about an unreachable child sitting in the corner all day banging his head. Just like Jimmy, he was always glued to his mother and had to be carried around the whole time to prevent endless crying. He also had no interest in toys or the environment, and I felt moved to read that the mother had also lost her friends and family relationships over her son's condition. It was overwhelming and shattering, and yet having a possible diagnosis opened up a whole new way forward for us.

Early Intervention

I talked to my friend Penny about my suspicions that Jimmy might be autistic, and she suggested right away that I call the early intervention program for children under three years of age. Jimmy's being under three meant I did not need a referral from my pediatrician, and also that I might qualify for help from a therapist.

Professionals state that there are three main reasons for early intervention with a child that either already has some developmental disability or is starting to show early signs of it:

1. To enhance the child's development
2. To provide support and assistance to the family
3. To maximize the child's and family's contribution to society

Researchers believe that human development is rapid in the pre-school years. It has been shown that early intervention is effective: children who received early intervention needed less special education and other services compared with children who did not receive such early treatments. Many professionals agree that treatment is most effective when the child receives 25 to 40 hours of therapy per week. Typically funding is available for behavioral therapy, physical therapy, speech therapy and sensory integration therapy. In most cases a team of professionals will evaluate the child and determine which service is appropriate.

But, of course at the time I called at the early intervention childhood center I knew nothing about any of the possibilities and had no idea what to expect. The receptionist was very friendly and non-judgmental, when I made an appointment to evaluate Jimmy's current social, physical and speech development. On the day of the evaluation I was filled with hope, feeling that surely we would at last get some help. A speech therapist, a physical therapist, and an occupational therapist showed up with a variety of toys. With Jimmy proceeding to scream for the entire duration of the visit, it soon became clear they would be unable to determine any of his skills and that they would have to rely solely on my descriptions of Jimmy's development. The visit was a disappointment.

When I brought up my suspicions that Jimmy might have autism, they just laughed at me. They did not believe that Jimmy had autism. They also dismissed Jimmy's speech delay and his physical and social challenges. I found this incomprehensible, as I knew that other babies were communicating with words while Jimmy just made sounds or screamed when he needed something. The speech therapist told me that the reason for Jimmy's lack of speech was that he was being raised bilingual. She decided that his social difficulties were just a result of his being a sensitive child.

I explained to the physical therapist that Jimmy was falling down a lot and that his body was really floppy. Her unsympathetic analysis was that Jimmy had no more challenges than other children and that I just needed to do my job as a mother. It seemed always to come back to the fact that I was simply a bad mother. Once again I was crushed. The one good outcome was that we would get occupational therapy for Jimmy's sensory integration problems and we got a referral to a social worker with whom I could talk about my parenting struggles.

I did not believe that occupational therapy alone would resolve Jimmy's challenges. I had no real idea how to get an autism diagnosis evaluation. I was all alone with my suspicions, and when I brought it up people thought I was out of my mind.

The occupational therapist came once a week for an hour but all she ended up doing was watch Jimmy screaming. I was hoping over time she would figure out how to work with him but all she did was sit on my couch doing nothing. I got frustrated and complained to the supervisor of early intervention. I could not accept that those professionals had no answers for me other than blaming me for my parenting skills.

The Small Miracle of the Wilbarger Brushing Protocol

As a result of this unhappy episode, I decided there was nothing for it but to take things into my own hands and find the answers myself. I began detailed online research, often staying up all night. From other parents I found out about the Wilbarger brushing protocol, invented by Patricia Wilbarger in 1991. This protocol for reducing sensory defensiveness should be carried out every two hours by a trained occupational therapist. Using a special surgical brush, deep pressure is applied to the skin on the arms, back, and legs. The stomach and the face are never brushed. After that, the child receives gentle compressions to the shoulders, elbows, wrists/fingers, hips, knees/ankles, and sternum. I read about how children very sensitive to touch just like Jimmy, were successfully treated with this technique.

I told my social worker about my discovery and I insisted that Jimmy needed an occupational therapist trained in this method. After two weeks, a new therapist called Melany arrived with the brush and showed me how to apply this protocol with Jimmy. As usual Jimmy just screamed when she came near him. I had to find a way to make him confortable around her. The only thing I could think of was gummy bears, which he loved very much. Every time she entered the house she would immediately give him some gummy bears. All she could do in the first session was to hand him gummy bears, but, slowly and very carefully in the second session she added some playful moments until he was ready to try the brush. After the first brushing she showed me how to do it, and I found that not only did it seem to work like magic, but that it was really easy to apply. He loved the gentle pressure of the brush, and the compressions and started crying less and smiling more.

Before the brushings he had always seemed tired. Now, he became more energetic, and for the first time I started taking him out to museums and parks. His body got so strong that he could run around for two hours at the park without falling down once. It was a joy to see this huge change in his energy level, but now that he cried a lot less, it became obvious that socially he acted very differently from other children his age. He ran around never checking where I was and never invited me to play with him. My suspicions that Jimmy had autism grew, and even though he appeared a lot happier, now I was actually more concerned that ever. I had to keep searching for clarity, even if it meant getting news that I didn't want to hear.

We Get the Autism Diagnosis

I decided to appeal to my social worker whose own child had autism. Surely she would be empathetic! I told her about my fears that Jimmy could well have autism and about how nobody believed me. Could she help me get an evaluation from an autism expert? I kept on insisting and she gave me the number of the director and leading autism expert at the autism center in our town. Finally, a real "professional" would assess our child. Hope surfaced again. Perhaps now we might really get the breakthrough we needed.

Two weeks later we went to the autism center where the director and a second therapist conducted an assessment. This consisted of both an evaluation of Jimmy and a thorough interview of the parents. Both professionals tried to engage Jimmy, but he kept moving away from them and was frightened by their attempts to play with him. He was always easily upset and overwhelmed. My husband and I could not stop talking, as we described everything we had been through. It was the first time we had felt really listened to, and this unaccustomed empathy moved us greatly. They seemed to really understand how difficult life had become for us. They were not surprised by anything we told them. They had seen it before.

Relief flooded my body and I almost felt I had arrived "home." I had been used to people blaming me or telling me I was just a first-time mother who didn't know what to do. After this almost cathartic and amazing session, they gave Jimmy an autism spectrum diagnosis.

It is not uncommon for parents whose child has been diagnosed with autism to feel a profound sense of loss, as they may have to give up the dreams they had for their child. Parents deal with this news in very different ways, and even within one family, reactions can be very different. While one parent might be paralyzed by the news and retreat into a private impenetrable grief, another parent might throw him or herself into frantic work, researching everything they can lay their hands on, or fill their days with desperate attempts to find a "cure." These divergences can lead to severe marital tensions. Precisely when parents need the most support, this is sometimes when they get the least from their partners. If such a situation continues, a dangerous gulf can open up between them that could even lead to separation.

What could help those hurting parents avoid such a tragic outcome? Joining a local autism support group could be constructive, as most people find sharing and empathizing with others in a similar situation to be therapeutic. Any sort of counseling may be productive, though, as in my own case, if the counselor has no idea about the particular kinds of stresses experienced by parents of autistic children, the help they offer might be limited.

The grieving may be intermittent, and some parents report never achieving closure in the grieving process. They might feel they have worked it all through and come to terms with the new reality but then discover that at times, such as on a child's birthday, they go through the grief all over again when they are hit once again with the recognition that their child is developmentally not as skilled as its peers. Given that the pressures at this time are very great, perhaps just knowing that these reactions are perfectly "normal" and very common might help couples be more inclined to seek help and prevent them from breaking apart.

The Swiss-born American psychiatrist Elisabeth Kübler-Ross (born 1926) pioneered the idea of providing psychological counseling to the dying, and the following model for processing grief is useful for anyone experiencing profound loss.

Processing Grief –The Kuebler- Ross Model

Some professionals apply the Kuebler-Ross Model (1969), which describes five stages of grief, after someone has lost a loved one or experienced some catastrophic loss. The stages are denial, anger, bargaining, depression, and acceptance. In the first stage, the person may deny the loss as a defense mechanism. During the second stage, the person may become angry about why this happened to them. In the third stage, the person acknowledges the fact of the condition, but hopes to change the outcome by a change of lifestyle or other actions such as appealing to a higher power. During the fourth stage, the person might isolate himself and spend most of the day crying. Finally, in the fifth stage, the person accepts his mortality, or that of a loved one, or other tragic event. Kuebler-Ross acknowledged that there are great variations amongst people, and that not everyone goes through all stages. Stages might be skipped or happen in a different order. Some people might get stuck at a stage or go through stages several times. It would be good to have scientific research on how this model applies to parents of autistic children.

I knew Jimmy was not a typical child, but even after the diagnosis I was still not fully convinced that he actually did have autism. Being so desperately in need of help, my first thoughts were that this diagnosis would be a way for us to finally get service and help from government agencies. I shared this reaction with family and friends, and added that probably after a few months of expert attention Jimmy would be fine. Everybody agreed. My husband could not accept that Jimmy had autism either but he was very happy we would finally get some support.

It seemed our whole family was in denial about the severity and impact of an autism diagnosis

My doubts about whether autism really was the right diagnosis drove me to keep on researching online. In most books autistic children were described as "being in their own world," and content when left alone. Jimmy on the other hand, needed to be with me all the time. Could it be that he actually had some different condition? On the other hand he was exactly like the boy I had found in the book.

I kept on reading, hoping for some clarity, and one day I came across the work of an impressive autism specialist called Steven Gutstein, who was the founder of RDI therapy. He emphasized that the autistic child lacks the ability to share his experiences with others, and usually communicates only for instrumental purposes. The autistic child will ask for things it wants like a cup of milk but will not share his day or a funny event with you. A constantly changing world is upsetting for most autistic children; they look for repetition instead of the excitement of novelty.

Gutstein points out that the fearful autistic child clings to its mother for instrumental purposes, for example, in our case we had developed a routine when Jimmy was distressed. Whenever this happened, he would cling to me because this routine was what he was used to. Gutstein's finding was quite a revelation to me, and his theories fitted Jimmy's behavior very well. I started realizing that Jimmy was indeed autistic, and that the chances were very small that he would ever find a job, get married or even live on his own. This recognition left me feeling as if I had been hit on the head by a hammer. I had a child with a developmental disability, and it would not go away with a couple of months of therapy. This was a lifelong condition. I cried and was angry with myself and the world. Why me?

It might seem odd, but my husband and my family did not understand why I was upset. They kept insisting everything would be just fine, which made me even more furious. I decided to ignore what they had to say, and after all my reading I knew what they didn't seem able to acknowledge.

It was painful to find my son's behaviors described in Gutstein's books and articles, but I knew it was essential that I learn much more about autism. I couldn't sit and cry forever. I needed to accept the diagnosis, but somehow I couldn't accept that he wouldn't be able to live a fulfilled and independent life. There was no time for a long grieving period. My son needed my help.

Trying Floortime Therapy

Although I was ready to explore Gutstein's RDI therapy, my social worker had recommended Floortime as an appropriate therapy since RDI seemed costly and was not funded by the state. Floortime Therapy was developed by Dr. Stanley Greenspan, for children with autism. His therapy model assumes there are six milestones of development. Those are self-regulation and interest in the world, intimacy, two-way communication, complex communication, pretended play, and emotional thinking. The goal of Floortime

Therapy is to achieve those milestones and it also recognizes that some autistic children have sensory problems.

In Floortime the child sets the tone and directs the play

In Floortime the therapist observes the child and determines how best to approach it. The child leads the play while the therapist provides systematic challenges. He or she opens and closes circles of communication with words or gestures. For example, the therapist smiles at the child, and it smiles back. With the child directing the play, it follows that this should be enjoyable.

My social worker recommended I read a book called "The Boy Who Loved Windows" which was written by the mother. The boy described was hypersensitive to the environment, and he socially isolated himself. Through intensive interventions including Floor time therapy as well as dietary changes, the boy transformed into a happy interactive child able to attend regular school. However I could not find any other recovery stories, though a lot of parents did describe Floortime as very helpful. They especially liked the aspect that it was a child-centered therapy allowing the child to be in control of the interactions. The fact that a lot of parents used Floortime therapy and that Jimmy could be in charge of the interactions seemed very attractive to me. Usually all the interactions I had with Jimmy happened on his terms, and he refused any of my play ideas. I was very happy to give Floortime a try.

We qualified for Floortime Therapy every day for about three hours except on weekends. The therapist came with a suitcase full of toys, and since he was very playful Jimmy seemed to enjoy the interactions with him. The therapy went well when he used number puzzles and letter puzzles, which were the only things Jimmy was interested in. Jimmy also needed to be in charge of the interaction, and he got very upset when the therapist added little challenges. Usually the session ended after forty-five minutes when Jimmy started falling apart and screaming.

After the session I had to rock him in a dark room to calm him down for an hour or two. I had hoped that Jimmy's language would start improving and that he would begin to play more like other children his age. We tried this therapy for several months, but I could not see much improvement. I talked to the supervising therapist about the lack of progress, and she remarked that Jimmy had a higher cognitive functioning than the other children they were working with. It became clear that we needed to look into different therapies.

ABA Therapy

My social worker suggested that I try another state-funded therapy called ABA (Applied Behavioral Analysis). I had read the book "Let me Hear Your Voice" by Catherine Maurice, whose two autistic children had recovered with ABA therapy. When the author wrote the book, much less was known about autism than today and many people believed that autism was caused by a distant, emotionally unavailable mother. That theme of blaming the mother kept resurfacing in my research! I was impressed how the author and her husband refused to accept that their daughter's condition could not improve.

They found out about ABA, hired a couple of therapists, and set up an intense home program for their child. Her daughter made excellent progress with ABA, and she was soon indistinguishable from her peers.

Later her second child was also diagnosed with autism and he too made remarkable progress with ABA. The book didn't go beyond childhood, and we don't know if these children show signs of autism as adults, or if they live independently, have a partner or a job. After reading this fascinating book, I decided to do some further research on ABA.

Ivar Lovaas, a doctor of Psychology, developed this therapy in 1960 at the University of California, Los Angeles (UCLA). ABA therapy is based on the idea that when people are rewarded for a behavior, they are likely to repeat that behavior.

ABA therapy is based on the idea that when people are rewarded for a behavior, they are likely to repeat that behavior.

In the1987 study, Lovaas found that with 40 hours ABA therapy per week nearly half of the children were able to complete normal first-grade classes and achieved normal intellectual and educational functioning by the end of first grade. ABA therapy works on social and behavioral skills, communication, academic, or any other challenges a child presents.

Lovaas emphasizes that an ABA program needs to be a comprehensive program where the child should be taught in every setting every available moment. Tabletop drills need to be mastered in natural situations at home and in school. Best results can be reached when trained and supportive people including parents, teachers, relatives, and even peers, implement the learned skill in varied settings.

I started reading on the Internet about the experiences and the progress of autistic children whose major therapy was ABA. It seemed to me that the children were able to memorize social phrases, but they were not able to build true friendships and be flexible in complex social situations. I didn't find evidence that children who did improve with ABA had mastered skills that would lead to an independent adult life.

I was fixed on the idea that my child should be able to have an independent life

I read that the majority of adults with autism need lifelong support. In most cases, families need to create a home-based plan, or select a program or facility that provides ongoing help. This was very discouraging, and I decided not to apply ABA as a major therapy for Jimmy. Instead, I was considering using ABA techniques for certain skills like potty training or dressing, where using reinforcements could be helpful. For me, it was important that Jimmy would be able to make a true friend.

Chapter Four

THE REVELATION of RDI

Relationship Development Intervention (RDI) was developed by Steven Gutstein. Gutstein had been leading social skills groups for autistic children using behavior modification but became dissatisfied with this approach on finding that no matter how hard he worked, none of the children had learned to be genuinely curious about other people's feelings. Generally, humans are both curious about, and concerned with, the feelings of others and it is through this ability we find ways to connect socially and form relationships. Relationships often change and fluctuate but these connections with other people are what sustain us and help carry us through our lives.

It could also be said that it is through relationships with others that we grow and evolve at a deep personal level. Certainly Gutstein regarded the lack of true relationships as the main deficit in autistic children, and was moved to search for solutions. He researched and analyzed a vast amount of material on normal child development that led eventually to his developing an intervention model (RDI) to help children have meaningful relationships with others.

Gutstein believes that children on the autism spectrum have deficits in emotion sharing, social referencing, flexible thinking, co-regulation, relational information processing, and foresight and hindsight. Social referencing allows the child to use a partner as a reference point to alter his own actions. For example, a child looks at his mother to establish whether a toy is safe, and acts based on the mothers response. Anticipating an exciting event together would be an example of emotion sharing. Flexible thinking enables the child to alter strategies and plans in a changing environment. Co-regulation allows the child to add variations and remain coordinated with a partner. For example, the child can add to the fun of the play, and can make sure he and his friend stay together. Relational information processing makes it possible to find solutions to problems that have no right or wrong answer. Foresight and hindsight demonstrate the ability to reflect on past experiences and anticipate future scenarios. Partners interact in a changing environment, and need to constantly take their partner's point of view into consideration and adjust their own actions. This represents a major challenge for children on the autism spectrum. They rely on very predictable scripts and roles and become incompetent and frustrated in a dynamic social world. RDI is not a static intervention model but keeps evolving as scientists make new discoveries about child development.

When I started with RDI it consisted of 28 stages building on one another based on the autism deficits, each of them containing specific skills, which the child needs to master. I would advise anyone interested in going more deeply into RDI to research the RDI website for ongoing changes and further information. In order to implement this therapy parents would need to read the books and get a consultant. This book is not intended as a RDI handbook, it is more a general introduction and an account of my personal experiences with it.

After my initial research into RDI I was very impressed with the ideas and concepts. I had a real feeling of confidence that this method could indeed help our son. Intellectually and emotionally it made sense. Although generally this work is done with the help of a consultant, I decided to try it on my own as RDI looked as if it could become rather costly. I started out by reading both of Gutstein's books where I found guidelines and activities that I could do with Jimmy.

One of the first things I implemented was changing how I talked to Jimmy. Instead of asking questions or putting demands on him, I made statements and gave him time to figure out how to solve problems.

To this end I used less imperative and more declarative language. Steven Gutstein prefers a 20/80 percent ratio. For example I would say, "I wish I had a cookie" instead of telling him to bring me a cookie. If he climbed on the table I would tell him that it didn't look safe instead of telling him to get off the table. Instead of saying "good job" I would say, "I love how you drew the sun." Praising a child might put pressure on him whereas personal statements make no demands. I would make flashcards with the demands I used often during the day, and come up with alternative comments and statements. Often I would only use nonverbal communication so Jimmy could watch my actions instead of listening to my words.

After I had got to the stage of mostly using non-demanding language, I slowed down our interactions and instead of rushing through the day, I gave him time to figure things out on his own. For example, if he spilled his milk I would say "oops" shrug my shoulders and look at the spill. I would give him time to think about the solution, instead of rushing in and cleaning up the mess. I started looking for teachable moments during the day, and paused and waited a lot. We would step out of the door without his jacket, then I would just pause and say 'oops, looks like you will be cold" to see if he put his jacket on. When we set the table I would purposely forget an item and say "something is missing" and wait to see if Jimmy could figure it out.

Bedtime became the most difficult time. I had established a routine that ended up being unhelpful, as Jimmy often would scream for an hour if anything changed in the routine. He loved music, and as part of the bedtime routine I had used a CD and played exactly the same three songs every night. This worked until the CD player broke one night. I also read him a story every night, but even the smallest variations could cause a huge upset. He would cry inconsolably if I happened to drop the book or was reading with a hoarse voice.

Gutstein suggested introducing patterns in the activities and slowly introducing small changes. He emphasizes that those changes needed to be productive. The parent should introduce productive uncertainty, enough changes to keep the child challenged but not overwhelmed. For example for a bedtime song we would sing "Row, row, row your boat" and sometimes we would row a little slower or faster, moving back and forth, but still following the same pattern of rowing. We might change the song a bit into "Row, row, row your ship" etc., but keep the basic lyrics and music the same.

I started to create moments of anticipation by adding small, fun surprises in our daily life. A good place for making changes was his room. To make those changes noticeable, I had to take everything off the walls and make his room as empty as possible. This was quite emotionally difficult as I had decorated his room when he was a baby, and had spent weeks on art projects to make it beautiful. I had put my whole soul into creating a special place for Jimmy, even designing a beautiful aquarium with paper fish of different colors. When I had to take everything down it felt symbolic -- I had indeed lost the son I was dreaming of. It was one of the saddest moments when I realized that along with the pictures I was removing, my former bright expectations for my child had to go as well.

I bought three different posters for the walls and changed their location randomly every night. I also changed which poster I would put up. Before Jimmy and I entered his room, I would pause and wait until he looked at me, and then I would make an exited face and say "surprise, surprise." We would enter the room and look at the poster. I needed to make sure that we always had a close connection so I would hold his hand, or if he would not let me I would pick him up.

At first he was upset about the changes but after a while he started enjoying those games and began sharing his excitement with me. I also put a different stuffed animal in the closet every day. He grew to love opening the closet with me, and soon we were sharing more and more smiles.

Sometimes I made surprise bags with little items in them, and would take one out after another with pauses and excited facial expressions. Eventually I would just hide things behind my back. Sharing such experiences is different from eye contact. In RDI the child will not be trained to look into a person's eyes, but rather it learns to get information from facial gazing and expressions. A child might be able to have great eye contact, but at the same time not be able to share excitement or recognize a smile as approval. I really liked that RDI addressed this challenge.

After six months doing RDI without a consultant I felt stuck, as the books and the Internet did not provide enough information for me to move ahead on my own. Progress was clear, as Jimmy had become more flexible, but I did not know where to go from there. I felt I needed some professional support, as he still was still not prepared to give himself over to my guidance. Paying for consultants was beyond our means as my husband was still a postdoctoral fellow on a modest salary, and I had no income as I had to stay at home with Jimmy.

Fortunately some online friends helped us through this dilemma by suggesting we call Maggie, a consultant-in-training who would charge less. It turned out she was amenable to negotiating an affordable plan for us, this enabling a move ahead into the next stage. The most expensive part of this next step seemed to be the assessment to see where on the spectrum Jimmy was with his skills. During the assessment Maggie set up a variety of fun exercises with beanbags, trucks, balls and puzzles for my husband and me to do with Jimmy. I was shocked how anxious Jimmy was. He whined and cried and constantly ran toward the door to get out of the room.

Maggie had given us certain tasks to establish which objectives Jimmy had mastered already, so it would be clear at what stage of the RDI training we should start. For example, we had to run towards beanbags or play ball back and forth. Jimmy did not manage to do one single activity with us. He only engaged when he was fully in control of the activity, for example when we were supposed to play ball he would grab the ball and run away. But he would never throw the ball back or let us chase him. Another activity was "follow my eyes to the prize." I was hiding a toy under one of three beanbags, and Jimmy was supposed to find it based on where I was looking. Instead he would just run towards the door crying to get out.

Getting Jimmy to Trust our Guidance

In a follow-up meeting Maggie showed us how to set up activities that would help Jimmy to develop trust in us, and accept our guidance. One of the most helpful things she taught us was setting up a circuit. She arranged several beanbags in a circle. The task was to clean the beanbags together. First we would have to spray the beanbags and then dry them. I guided Jimmy from beanbag to beanbag holding hands. I gave him the spray bottle and let him make the beanbags wet. After a couple of rounds we would dry them. Maggie advised adding little variations such as hopping in between the beanbags or moving faster and slower. While we were cleaning the beanbags I would chant, "we are cleaning, we are cleaning" to make this activity more exciting.

This kind of activity worked very well, and Jimmy started to accept me as a guide. Maggie emphasized that a circuit made the task for Jimmy more predictable. That way he would be more willing to accept me as a guide and be in a master/apprentice relationship which was one of the foundations to build trust. We kept doing more exercises in a circuit during the assessment and though Jimmy stopped running away, by the end of the RDI assessment we found out that he had not mastered even the basic stages of RDI. We would have to work further with him on establishing the Master/Apprentice relationship first before working on other objectives.

My task was to work with Jimmy on activities throughout the day and send videos of it to Maggie. She would give me feedback, guide me through the challenges, and show me how to get to the next level in RDI. We decided to do most of our communication with videos and phone conferences since she lived quite a distance away. I would send her a video and call her every two weeks.

At home I would do very simple activities in circuits. Obviously it was best to start out with things that Jimmy liked to do, such as painting. I arranged pieces of paper in a circle and we would walk together painting on the pieces of paper as we went around. The important thing was that I stayed in charge of all the material, only handing paintbrushes to him when it was time to paint. I kept everything very simple, encouraging him to move on as soon as something was on the paper, for example, just a circle or even a line.

I gave him different colors and shapes to paint and also changed how we were moving. The changes might be pausing, dropping a paintbrush or spinning in a circle while we were walking. I watched Jimmy closely so as not to overwhelm him with the variations. After eight weeks of doing such activities Jimmy was well on his way to being a good apprentice. I could add new activities and expand old ones. He became more motivated to play instead of wanting to run away. His developing trust in me as a guide opened the door for us to begin an RDI lifestyle.

We Begin an RDI Lifestyle

To expose Jimmy to new environments I would take him out every day to stores I thought he would like. This was not at all about shopping, but allowing me to be in control as his guide, holding his hand and leading him from store to store to new discoveries. Sometimes I would pause or walk a little slower or faster, sometimes I would walk backwards. I kept the store visits very short. I would point out a couple of objects but then move on quickly so that Jimmy would not get too focused on any items. I opened up a new world for him without overwhelming him. We visited pet stores, cafés, grocery stores and hardware stores. Although I was certain these exercises were going to be extremely valuable, those outings were far from easy.

Often Jimmy resisted staying with me, and it was hard for me to hold onto a screaming child in public. When we took walks in the neighborhood, at the beginning he would just lie down on the sidewalk and refuse to get up. Rather than forcing him to get up, I would just hold his hand and wait until he was ready to get up. This could take thirty minutes or longer, and I just had to ignore neighbors and strangers staring at us.

I remember once I let him walk by himself because the constant struggle was just too much. On that occasion he ran right into a busy street. A stranger caught him and yelled at me, leaving me feeling incompetent and judged. Again! I had had years of feeling criticized and judged, and this was always hard to bear. In my reading I saw that so many mothers of autistic children got messages from the people around them, including professionals, that they were simply inadequate parents. It is quite tragic to think of those mothers wrestling with lives that had become almost impossible, trying with all their might to somehow find a way to help their child, and on top of all that to have to bear criticism and judgment.

Fortunately over time Jimmy got used to holding my hand, and if he tried to get away from me I would simply switch hands, pick him up or give him a piggyback ride to add changes. The object was to always keep him close to me. It remained challenging, and I wondered if he would ever just comfortably walk next too me. This almost seems funny now, as these days he loves to hold my hand and do things with me.

Cooking, Cleaning and Artwork

At home we started doing activities that gave us a good framework for RDI exercises such as cooking, cleaning, laundry and artwork. I would hand him the cooking ingredients and we would stir together. We did dusting together, filled up the washing machine, and we did lots of artwork. I always needed to add enough uncertainty to keep Jimmy motivated to watch me.

I varied the way I did things, and sometimes handed him things slowly or fast, up high or down low. I made Jimmy laugh by mixing in items that didn't belong, and kept him involved by throwing or hiding things. I would pretend to be sleeping, hide under a beanbag or run away to see if he would get me back into the game. I would make mistakes; break things; sometimes pretend to cry or fall down to see if he was able to repair the action.

Soon I was doing RDI everywhere. I would fall down on the sidewalk to see if he would help me up. I dropped my key on the sidewalk to see if Jimmy noticed. Things would fall out of my hands while I was shopping. Spilling the coffee in the café gave an opportunity for us to clean it up together. I even knocked down a board game while playing, and then acted as if it wasn't a big deal – "oops, anther mistake".

We would play with balloons in the café and do the laundry at the Laundromat, pretending our washing machine was broken. I would rip a magazine so we could fix it together. Crazy cloth bought together at the thrift store was perfect for dress up parties at home. We did odd things like drinking out of bowls and eating popcorn with spoons: sometimes we would eat under the table and sleep in sleeping bags in the living room. We were dancing and spinning together. Those moments of pure fun were very precious to me after all the hard times we had had before.

Finding Inspiration in Stores

Being all day with Jimmy I was constantly searching for new ideas for playing with him. Many of the big box stores were a godsend and provided much inspiration. We found great activities in the seasonal section, and among the toys, clothes, and bikes. The staff let us try every possible item. Jimmy actually learned to ride his bike without training wheels at one of the stores. Of course we went at the time when the store was empty.

Mattress stores were favorite destinations on rainy days. We pretended we wanted to buy a mattress, and had fun hopping from one bed to the next. We lay down or jumped together to see which bed was the biggest, softest or the most comfortable. Sometimes we pretended being asleep and waking each other up. In Boston's, extreme weather, we were thankful for those great indoor places where we could do RDI as we tried skateboards, footballs, basketballs and soccer balls.

I am very aware that not everyone is able to stay home with their autistic child. Many parents have so much economic pressure that both are obliged to work. If parents have several children to take care of, it is difficult to give so much time to just one child. In the case of a single parent it must be particularly hard. Some parents involve other family members such as grandparents or older siblings to implement RDI at home, while others train a babysitter and caretakers in daycare or school settings. However, parents should ideally be very involved as the primary caretaker implementing RDI in daily life. Every day they need to set aside special time to concentrate on their autistic child. Almost every activity can offer an opportunity for the child to act as an apprentice. The task can be as simple as coloring, mopping the floor or just taking a short walk outside.

My video camera was always with me when we went out, as I had to record the activities I did with Jimmy for the RDI consultant. I had to learn how to film Jimmy and myself at home, outside and in stores. Sometimes I asked permission to film and other times I just put the camera on the shelf of the store. Outside I would put the camera on the car, on stairs, on the sidewalk or I would bring cardboard boxes to put the camera on.

In cafés I would only go when it was not crowded so I could cover the camera with a small towel, and put it on the table next to us or on the stroller. Filming was quite challenging, since I not only had to work with Jimmy, but also make sure we both were filmed and that the camera didn't get stolen.

Our consultant recommended making memory books to spotlight the things we were working on. I took pictures of us both while we were doing RDI to highlight the important part of the interaction. Together we put the pictures in a book, and I wrote underneath each picture what needed to be highlighted. Those were very short phrases such as "oops" or "we did this together." We would not focus on the objects in the picture, but highlight the experience.

While shopping I took pictures of the produce, as it was fun to show Jimmy a photo of the item we would buy next. Often I would mix in a picture of his dad, an animal or myself to make him laugh. The store manager did not think that was very funny, and once he even asked me to leave, as he didn't want their produce to be photographed. In spite of occasional opposition I managed to do what I had to do. I wanted my son to get better, and I was very determined.

Beginning to Play with other Children

The Children's Museum and the Science Museum also offered good play places. It was important to avoid big crowds, so we usually went on Mondays when we had those places practically to ourselves. Jimmy was still afraid of children at times, and I had started giving him a gummy bear every time he was close to a child or a child approached him. He still had plenty of meltdowns when we could not avoid a crowd.

I was not sure if he would ever be able to play with another child. Gradually he stopped panicking around other children but he never made an attempt to initiate play or respond to an invitation to play, and he still continued to mostly tune out other people.

When Jimmy was about three and a half years old a fortunate opportunity presented itself when a couple with a four year old son moved in next door. I remember clearly the first time he met the new boy. He whined and hid behind my legs when the boy tried to initiate play. As his mom and I soon became friends, I decided to ask her if I could "borrow" her son to have a play date with Jimmy. She was completely in favor of this as it gave her some free time for herself.

According to the RDI plan Jimmy was not supposed to play with other children yet, but I wanted him to start getting used to other kids as soon as possible. I set up activities like play dough, stamping or rice play. Initially they didn't interact much with each other, and I often had to rescue Jimmy from being too overwhelmed by the other boy. I kept these play dates to thirty minutes or less. Over time Jimmy showed more and more interest in playing with the other boy and eventually they started running, biking and riding their scooters together. It felt as if we were suddenly in a very different place. It did take almost a year for this to happen, but it was nonetheless an amazing achievement.

For the first time I was able to hang out with another mom while our kids were playing. It sounds like such a simple everyday thing but I had seriously wondered if this would ever happen. I could not keep my eyes off Jimmy playing away so happily and enjoying his new independence. All that work had paid off. We even went on to spend the holidays with the boy's family.

When Christmas came around it marked the first time Jimmy was out of my lap. While all the adults were sitting and finishing their Christmas dinner, the kids started playing on the floor. This was the first time I had finished a holiday meal since Jimmy was born. I was ecstatic and very hopeful for the future. Things that other people took for granted were, for me, like small wonders and gifts to be savored.

Options for Families with Several Children

In bigger families siblings can take over the role of a peer or a playgroup situation. Parents can offer music, art time or reading time for all children in a more structured setting to avoid their autistic child getting overwhelmed. Also parents could get all siblings involved in household tasks: the important thing is to give each child a role they are competent in. For example, a two year old could hand the mother the laundry, while a six year old could sort it and the twelve year old could fold it. Everybody could go on a walk together looking at flowers, rocks and collecting leaves. Families can take all kids to a less crowded park and play an obstacle course or swing together. Parents or siblings might have to hold their autistic child's hand to keep her/him calm and focused. Siblings can be excellent playmates for their autistic brother or sister.

Implementing RDI in a Playgroup

When Jimmy became more confident in the German playgroup I had set up, I decided to make this group more RDI friendly. Being the leader and in charge of the program, I was able to implement RDI in the songs and games, and also during organized playtime. I often used nursery rhymes they knew and would make funny changes in the lyrics.

Soon the children had fun coming up with their own variations. Jimmy became excellent at this over time, amazing me by how many song variations he could invent. I brought music that the children could dance to, or they happily played along with different instruments. Jimmy liked the German group and never missed a song.

Once he had mastered coordinating his movements with mine, he amazed me by starting to play with the others during the free time part of the German group. He started running around with the other children, playing chase and hide and seek. Then one day he spontaneously joined into a noisy rumbustious game where the children were all on top of each other in a parachute being moved around by some parents. Only a month before this my son could not even bear to be in the room with another child, and here he was now sitting in the middle of a bunch of screaming kids having just as much fun as them. It seemed we were now at least part of the way "out of the woods".

Not everybody will be able to set up and lead a group. Community centers and private organizations offer playgroups for children. It is up to the parent to find an appropriate setting. Professionals can make suggestions but parents have to ensure that their child is not overwhelmed in special needs groups or other social activity groups. Obviously, it's really important that your child likes the activities. Lots of children like music and dance because it offers some predictability. In general, smaller groups of three to five children are preferable. Notice if the group is well organized or mostly chaotic. Observing the group carefully will help you determine if the setting is right for your child's age, interests and ability to function in a group setting.

Travelling with Jimmy

Seeing Jimmy's great progress in RDI and his improved confidence in groups, I agreed to a trip across the country to visit my husband's grandmother and uncle. I still was very nervous about this, since Jimmy still required a lot more attention than other kids his age. I was worried that my husband's family would blame me for Jimmy's issues, as so many other people had done. Fortunately my anxieties proved groundless, as they were completely supportive. They celebrated Jimmy, and reassured me that I was a great mother – something I always wanted to be.

The visit went so well that my husband suggested a trip to Germany to see my family. Jimmy did amazingly well with all the changes that faced him in Germany, though he still was not open to interacting with his grandparents. It was hard for my parents to see their grandson was afraid of them. They both seemed worried and clearly saw that he was not the typical child. They kept commenting on how Jimmy did not explore their beautiful yard or their house. Instead Jimmy stayed glued to me or to my husband during the entire trip.

However, I still regarded it as a huge success, as just one year earlier I would not have even dreamt that such a trip would be possible. RDI had helped us to open up Jimmy's world and also to reunite with our families.

Which Intervention is Best?

RDI is no magic bullet, and although I don't think RDI "cures" autism, it can bring about a vast and liberating improvement in quality of life for both the child and the parents. Without any doubt at all, our life was transformed by RDI and it enabled our son to successfully form real friendships and relationships of many kinds. I will always be so very thankful for the people who supported me in choosing to live an "RDI lifestyle". There are a lot of parents who had success with Floor time, ABA or other approaches or combinations of therapies. Each family has to decide what is best for them and their child in their specific situation. I do not believe there is one solution appropriate for everyone.

Chapter Five

THROUGH REGRESSION TO NEW HOPE

Finding a Biomedical Treatment

The Dramatic Regression

Jimmy's crash back into severe autism right before his 4th birthday came as a shock -- especially after all the good progress with the RDI treatment! He had progressed to the stage of enjoying simple games with me, but now when I tried to play with him he started crying and moving away. The dramatic relapse came at the time I was weaning him off breast milk. At the beginning of this process it didn't really register that Jimmy had become more tired and less playful but when I was down to one feeding a day it became disturbingly evident. Not only did he start crying a lot more, but also he became strangely depleted of all energy. For example when I took him to a store he refused to walk or even stand up, and just lay down on the floor looking completely exhausted. His anxiety level skyrocketed at that time and again he refused to play with other children. This meant the end of the happy play dates with the neighbor's boy. It was profoundly dispiriting – like a door slamming in our faces.

His language regressed dramatically. He stopped pointing things out or telling me what he had done – all declarative language was gone, and in fact, all meaningful language started to disappear. His verbal communication regressed into repetitive counting or asking the same meaningless question over and over. He would spend long periods of time playing with his fingers, waving them in the air or kneeling down on the wooden floor pressing his hands into the cracks of the wood. Often he stared mesmerized at the cracks. Other times he would just spin around endlessly.

The terrible 4.30 a.m. waking up now also started again! If I was really lucky I could sometimes get him to sleep until 5 am. It was so upsetting to see him in the early morning walking listlessly in a weird sort of slow motion, like someone in a drunken stupor. He would barely eat anything other than fish sticks or water popsicles. (Popsicles seemed to be the one thing that could sometimes calm him down in a long crying episode). What was wrong with him?

Even his drawing skills vanished and he started crying when he realized he was unable to even hold a marker anymore. His teeth turned dark, no matter how much I brushed them. He had changed into an unhealthy and sad looking child. The mirror showed me that I wasn't looking much better myself. Stress and lack of sleep were taking their toll on both of us.

This relapse affected everything and in the German playgroup things went downhill as well. Jimmy's anxiety was so high that he started clinging and crying when any child approached him. During the sing-along he sat there completely unresponsive, picking strings from the carpet with his fingers. Even when someone called his name to join in the songs there was no response at all. Music had always been one of his favorite things, but now he didn't seem to even be aware of it. During snack time he would often fall off the chair, unable even to sit up. His being there was clearly pointless, and I had no other choice but to leave this group we both had loved so much.

His separation anxiety became so intense that I was unable to spend any time apart from him. I stopped even taking the trash out. He would scream and cry if I tried to go out the front door. He would not even stay with my husband anymore. Much of his days were spent sitting and staring blankly into nothingness. I continued to feel how peculiar it was that he seemed to absolutely need my close proximity even though he was not truly interacting with me.

I sent my RDI consultant a video. She was shocked that Jimmy had slipped back so much, and could not believe how autistic he looked. After our huge relief at the recent progress, this sudden downward spiral was almost unbearable.

Unraveling Under the Stress of Jimmy's Decline

Day after day I had to helplessly watch him going downhill. No RDI therapy could help him now. I still don't know how I survived those long months stuck at home. I found myself crying helplessly on the phone when I tried to tell anyone who called about what was going on. I think I was beginning to have a sort of breakdown, and I cried often and easily. The truth was I felt as if I was falling apart. My family and my friends got tired of me. It went so far that we agreed I would not answer the phone anymore. I was no fun to be around, and people asked me to stop being so negative and pessimistic. I tried hard to fulfill people's expectations but I just could not.

I felt alone and very depressed to the point that I could no longer go on living under those conditions. This was a real crisis, and some radical action was called for. I had always thought I had the power to change my life. But now I was losing my son in front of my eyes and there was nothing I could change about that. I could not rip out the pain and there was no escape. Reluctantly, I decided to go on anti-depressants. I told my doctor of my plight and my decision, and I refused the talk-therapy he offered. I did not want to hear that I needed to accept my son as he was. The anti-depressants made things a little bit more bearable, and took the edge off my pain. I cried less and at least now I was able to function somewhat in daily life.

Considering Desperate Measures

Jimmy's separation anxiety was so great that I found myself resorting to bribery -- but not even the promise of getting the best candy would budge him. I became desperate to find new ways of making progress. I even thought about putting him on psychiatric medication. He was only three and a half, and it broke my heart that I had to even consider this.

I talked to one mom who had given her son anti-depressants at the age of eight because she had no other choice. Her son had become very aggressive and was also unable to separate from her. Jimmy hadn't shown any aggression so far but the crying and anxiety reminded the other mom of her son. She said, "You are the first mom I ever met who has a similar story." Anti-depressants can have side effects for children and especially teenagers, so she advised me to do thorough research. Apparently some teenagers on anti-depressants have committed suicide. In her case though, the anti-depressant turned out to be a lifesaver. Her son's aggression and anxiety slowly started to disappear. After living for many years in a kind of prison with her son, the medication gave everybody in the family a new life. She later took him off the medication when he was a teenager and he continued to do well. I gritted my teeth and called several child psychiatrists thinking that perhaps this could help us too. It turned out that none of them was available and the waiting lists were ridiculous. I had no idea that it would be so difficult to meet with a child psychiatrist!

Dead Ends and Frustration

With Jimmy still screaming and crying hysterically if I was out of sight even for a moment, I absolutely had to get some sort of help. As he was constantly glued to me, I could barely do even the simplest tasks. Cooking and cleaning became impossible. By now he was over three and a half years old and he was getting taller and heavier. Often my back hurt so badly that I could only crawl through the house. I decided to call the autism specialist who had given Jimmy the original diagnosis. Surely she could help in some way. I wanted to ask her for an anxiety disorder diagnosis, hoping this would make us eligible for help from the State. Maddeningly, in spite of many attempts to reach her I never heard back.

Back at square one again I reflected that I couldn't be the only mother in this situation, so I hunted on the internet and found a support group for parents whose children had anxiety disorders. Sadly, that also was a dead end. After a lot of discussions it became clear that these parents were no further ahead than I was. I was surprised and disheartened to see that even with medications and therapy, the majority of these children had not improved.

Friends and family members kept insisting that Jimmy just had to get used to being separated from me and that I needed to hire a babysitter. When I found Wattana, a lovely girl with endless patience, I thought I would give this a shot. She was very experienced with special needs children, and I loved her gentle way of approaching Jimmy. We decided she should first spend time with Jimmy when I was present, and then I would leave the house for ten minutes. I could see Wattana had great talent at engaging children. Even if he was not at all not interested in playing, to my surprise she did manage to get a smile out of him. After two meetings I left the two of them alone for the first time. It was like torture to keep on walking, as I could hear his high-pitched screaming from a block away. When I came home Jimmy looked completely exhausted and he held out his little arms to me, clinging on for dear life.

Wattana told me his behavior was of great concern to her but she agreed to keep on trying. She had hoped the screaming would stop after a couple of weeks. Weeks passed and turned into months. I spent a lot of money on flowers and chocolate to show our great appreciation, and to encourage her to keep trying to help our son. We tried shorter absences and longer ones. We tried cookies, videos and music but Jimmy kept on crying and screaming. In all those months he never managed to stop once. After six months I had to let this kind babysitter go. I told other mothers about my experience and they warned me that not every babysitter might be as patient as her. They had heard of high-need children being abused by their babysitter. Not wanting to risk this, I decided not to hire anyone else.

Trying a Gluten and Casein Free Diet

With no help forthcoming from professionals or support groups, I once again returned to searching in bookstores as, after all, this had brought me to the first breakthrough in autism. I was driven by the thought that the answer had to be written down somewhere, and indeed soon I did discover a book that made a great impression on me. It described an autistic boy who recovered from autism by changing his diet. The idea that there could be a diet/autism connection had never entered my mind.

After reading this, Jimmy's dramatic regression after I stopped breastfeeding him, suddenly made sense. It was very interesting to learn that eating gluten (found in wheat products) and casein (found in dairy products) could lead to autistic behavior. The boy's mother also described that her son had lots of bacterial issues such as yeast in his gut. She claimed that her son recovered when she eliminated gluten and casein from his diet as well as giving him supplements and anti-yeast medication. This case was quite inspiring, so I bought the book and two days later I searched the stores for gluten and casein free items to try the diet with Jimmy. I also eliminated all sugars as I learned that sugar could feed the "bad" bacteria in the gut.

Astonishingly, within two weeks Jimmy started to change to the extent that he began playing with his fire truck and two little play dolls. As I had never seen him doing this before, I could hardly believe my eyes. I was so excited that I grabbed the camera and started filming him. I could not wait to show my husband the good news! He was surprised but very doubtful that eliminating gluten could have such a big impact on Jimmy's behavior.

Keeping him on this diet though, was extremely hard. I made my first mistake by unknowingly giving him a cookie containing gluten, and the reaction started within two hours. It turned out that even tiny crumbs or even gluten dust could cause a reaction. Even with the smallest gluten contamination all his language improvement disappeared and he became very spaced out. Back came the old frightening autistic behaviors such as sitting staring at the floor touching the cracks over and over, or playing with his fingers in front of his face. Once more he was gone, and this time it was worse than ever before with the crying and absurdly early waking returning as well. It was evident he was in pain, and that the food sensitivities were a central issue, so I was deeply disturbed that it wasn't possible to make this diet work! When we went away for several days at a time it was especially difficult to follow through with it.

I remember one trip to California when we went with my husband on a business trip. I had prepared gluten and dairy free food to take with us, but feeding Jimmy in a hotel without a stove or fridge was no easy matter. I was extremely careful not to contaminate Jimmy's food, and made sure not even a crumb of gluten or dairy passed his lips. In spite of all these efforts he still regressed on the third day, again becoming obsessed with the cracks in the hotel floor. I was highly frustrated when I found out that the hotel soap contained gluten. After all the care I had taken! I felt I could not win this battle, as those substances seemed to be hidden in just about everything: play dough, soap, shampoo, meats, juices, breads and so many more items.

I hated this diet because no matter how hard I tried it was impossible to be successful. I also suspected that Jimmy had other food sensitivities as well, so I rotated his foods and kept a diary to find out what exactly was causing him trouble. Unfortunately I could not come to any definite conclusions. He was not getting better, and indeed he was actually getting worse. He had changed so positively at the beginning of the new diet that now I felt frustrated and very disappointed. What on earth could I do now?

Further digging on the Internet turned up some support groups who suggested that the diet might work better if I gave Jimmy vitamins and minerals. I ordered multivitamins, calcium, magnesium, vitamin B12 and pro-biotics and gave him these supplements one at a time, beginning at a very low dose. Those vitamins seemed to make his symptoms worse even at the lowest doses. He either cried or got more spaced out. Desperately, I posted messages asking for help and advice on every possible Internet autism site. Nobody had answers for me.

The Question of Vaccinations

The next glimmer of light came about a month later when I had a phone call from a friend who told me about a highly recommended homeopathic pediatrician. I didn't know much about homeopathy though I was aware that it had a large following in Germany and some other countries. Basically homeopaths believe the body heals itself when the patient takes minute quantities of the same substances originally causing the illness. As this branch of alternative medicine has been around for several hundred years and has many dedicated followers, I thought it could be worth taking my friend's advice. I was very daunted by the prospect of a two-hour train ride to the doctor's office since such trips were usually a great ordeal.

Jimmy was such an attractive little boy that people often tried to interact with him or even touch him, something that could bring on a screaming episode. There were no elevators at the train station but I declined all offers of help with carrying the stroller up the stairs, fearing this could set him off again. On top of this he hated being confined to a stroller on the platform. Everyone could see me struggling to prevent him from running on the train tracks. It was a wonder no one accused me of child abuse, hearing my son's hysterical screams. Somehow we did manage to get to the doctor's office. I was very amazed at her empathetic and warm personality. This was the first time a medical professional had showed real concern and interest in our predicament. She had only ever seen one other child with autism before but she was eager to learn all about Jimmy's history. Her major interest was in his vaccinations. She believed that some of them, and especially those containing the neuro-toxin mercury, could be harmful to the child's brain development. She asked me to find out if any of Jimmy's shots had contained mercury, and she also wanted to know about the behaviors he was presenting at the time he was vaccinated. She believed there could be an autism-vaccine connection.

I hated going back to my old pediatrician's office remembering the unfriendly receptionist who thought I was just a hysterical mother who had nothing better to do than complain about her child. At first she refused to help me, but I insisted I needed to see Jimmy's old vaccination records. I was just on the verge of shouting at her when she went and consulted my old pediatrician.

I didn't expect him to be cooperative but to my surprise he was very open and told me he wanted to help me as much as he could. Apparently all of Jimmy's DTaP vaccines (diphtheria, pertussis, tetanus) had contained mercury. I was shocked. I had not expected this, and I had no idea that vaccines contained mercury. If only I had known then that vaccines without mercury were available! The idea of a neurotoxin being put in my baby's little body was deeply upsetting. I wish I had researched this whole topic beforehand and been able to discuss the options with the doctor.

I made a list of all the autistic behaviors and the times of each vaccine. Seeing it all written down I began wondering if there could be a possible link between the vaccinations and Jimmy's symptoms. He was vaccinated against Hepatitis B, Rotavirus, Whooping Cough, Tetanus, Diphtheria, Flu, Pneumococcal bacteria, Polio, Measles, Mumps, Rubella, and Varicella. He had his last DTaP at nineteen months when one of the biggest regressions had occurred. Could that be just a coincidence? After the MMR (measles, mumps, rubella) vaccine he had stopped gaining weight and developed on-going diarrhea. I was curious to see what research articles had found.

The majority of the research showed no link between autism and vaccines. There was one study by the British physician Andy

Wakefield, who enjoyed some popularity with parents of autistic children, indicating that the MMR vaccine might contribute to the development of autism in certain children. The General Medical Council, Britain's medical regulator, concluded later on that Andrew Wakefield's research was unethical since he failed to disclose payments from lawyers representing parents who believed the MMR vaccine had brought on autistic reactions. Also they regarded the study as unscientific as the sample pool was too small. The publishing journal then retracted the research paper and Dr Wakefield lost his medical license.

I could not find any articles confirming a direct connection between mercury and autism. Mercury is known to be toxic to the brain and clearly a lot more research needs to be done in this area. Researchers need to look at all the vaccines and the combinations of the vaccines given, as well as the individual predisposition of a child to develop autism. I think that today if I had to have a second child vaccinated, as a precaution I would only do it when it was healthy, and I would spread the vaccinations further apart, not giving multiple shots at one time.

I went back to the doctor's office with my paperwork. Hearing that the biggest regression had occurred after the DTaP shot, she ended up recommending a DTaP remedy. I administered this over many months, but unfortunately I could not see a significant improvement. I had really hoped that homeopathy might be the answer. It was very hard but in spite of all the promising possibilities that didn't lead to real break-throughs, in spite of all the hard disappointments, I never for a moment thought of giving up on the quest for solutions. It was not an option, since accepting Jimmy's condition would be accepting that he would never be able to play, learn or have a happy childhood. He was still sick and totally unable to do what other children could do.

Trying Other Alternative Approaches

Around that time a mother of an autistic child contacted me. She was interested in the RDI treatment I had been doing with Jimmy and in our conversations I recounted my sorry tale of all the unsuccessful treatments I had tried. Apparently her own son had been afflicted with severe crying spells as an infant and these had been completely resolved after treatment from a Kinesiologist. He had tested her son's food sensitivities and molds in the gut by muscle testing, and advised her to remove those foods from her son's diet.

Afterwards, I found out that applied Kinesiology works under the assumption that every organ dysfunction is accompanied by a specific muscle weakness, and muscle testing is used as a tool to diagnose body dysfunctions. Many people think that muscle testing for food sensitivities is impossible, and it needs to be done by laboratory tests. Honestly, the method did not make much sense to me, but as nothing so far had been really successful, I put my skepticism aside and decided to give this a try. I made an appointment with a kinesiologist and the day soon came when I packed some toys and snacks and off we went.

Discovering Food Sensitivities

When the doctor appeared, he welcomed us in such a warm manner that I felt very comfortable with him. Although the diagnostic process was very time consuming, he knew exactly how to engage a child in a playful way, and I marveled at how Jimmy sat still and cooperated throughout it all. He had to hold each of the eighty vials of different food substances while lifting his arm, so the doctor could test the weakness of the arm muscle. It turned out that he had about twenty food sensitivities and several molds in his gut.

After this rather unusual one and a half hour session, we left his office with some grapefruit seed extract and apple-cider vinegar for the molds. I needed to keep him off all the foods he was sensitive to including wheat, dairy, corn, some vegetables and some fruits. Within three days Jimmy stopped crying and turned into a happier and more active child. I will never forget the day he pointed out the moon to me. He even regained his drawing skills. One day I took Jimmy to visit my husband at work. Usually I avoided taking him there as he would be very anxious, clingy and withdrawn, but this time he surprised us. Not only did he draw a beautiful picture for one of the staff members but he also had a conversation with her about it. This had never happened before! This was the breakthrough we hadn't dared to believe would happen. This doctor was my hero!

Gluten Wars

Even though this treatment was so successful I was frustrated that the food sensitivities were changing constantly, and that Jimmy remained sensitive to gluten and casein. This required us to see this new doctor every three weeks even though we could barely afford it, and my husband was far from convinced this was a viable treatment. When Jimmy had a gluten infraction he would still revert to seeming very autistic. It was therefore essential to continue with this difficult diet as best I could. It was clear that Jimmy was feeling much better when he was not eating the offending foods but in spite of this, some of my family pressured me to stop this diet. They could not accept that gluten sensitivity existed and they accused me of malnourishing my child. I felt as if I was on a perpetual battlefield. I knew in my heart that gluten made Jimmy sick so I insisted on keeping to it. At this point he was only able to eat about ten foods, and although he had less pain, it was very exhausting for me to be constantly justifying the extremely limited diet. I persevered with it, but knew it couldn't be the full answer to his autism puzzle.

Chelation Therapy

I started to read about other treatments, and became interested in chelation therapy. The idea is that some children have a lot of harmful metals such as mercury and lead in their bodies. A chelator like EDTA (ethylenediaminetetraacetic acid) or DMSA (dimercaptosuccinic acid) binds the metal in the body and the body excretes the metals through urine or stool. There were a lot of websites about groups of parents who tried this kind of treatment. As with any other method, for some it seemed to work while for others it didn't. In some cases the children actually got worse. I could not find any scientific evidence that chelation could indeed help autism. Many articles emphasized that chelation could be a risk for children's health. I was shocked to read that a five-year-old boy had died while being given an intravenous injection of EDTA. This illustrates just how careful parents need to be when treating their children bio-medically.

Further research led me to information about a chelation protocol created by Andy Cutler. He had studied chemistry, and he himself had suffered from mercury poisoning. Many parents trusted his chelation protocol. He claims that children benefit mostly when DSMA is administered every eight hours based on the child's weight. I was very curious to learn more about this protocol and I ordered both of his books.

After reading them, I decided it was safe to go ahead and try this protocol with Jimmy. There are a lot of different chelating protocols but Andy Cutler always emphasized only using tiny amounts of the chelator to make sure the process is safe. I started giving Jimmy these tiny amounts of DMSA every eight hours. It was difficult to wake up him up in the middle of the night to give him pills but my hopes were high that I would see the same progress that some other parents had reported after only a few rounds of treatment. Perhaps this was going to be the thing that would make all the difference. It turned out to be another blind alley though, and after some time I had to accept that this was bringing no significant progress and I had to give it up. By this time I had tried so very many treatments but a real solution seemed maddeningly elusive.

I learned that not all children responded to the same treatment in the same manner. Unfortunately I was not one of the lucky ones whose child recovered by just doing a gluten free diet. I was not the lucky one whose child showed amazing progress after the first two rounds of chelation. Why was it so difficult for us to make any steady progress when so many other people did? It was hard to take – and hard to remain optimistic!

I spent every waking moment obsessively reading and searching on the Internet. As I didn't know what else to do, I did continue doing the RDI treatment though Jimmy was not making much progress with it during that time. I also kept going to the Kinesiologist in spite of feeling we were probably just treating the symptoms. The anti-depressants helped me through the worst times but often I would be overtaken by gloom, and would call my husband at work telling him that it looked as if I had better accept that we had an autistic child that might never live independently, have friends or have a job. I tried to accept that one day he might have to live in an institution, but deep down I could absolutely not come to terms with Jimmy being stuck with a life like that.

By now I had become so run down that I also had developed food sensitivities. The permanent stress led to a profound all consuming exhaustion. Some days I felt so completely worn out that I had trouble even getting out of bed. I saw my family practitioner but he just commented that when people get older they don't feel so good anymore. Older? I wasn't even forty yet. I wanted him to test me for food sensitivities but he refused to do so. The constant humidity in Boston just made things worse.

The Difficulty of Maintaining Balance in Marriage

Not surprisingly, I had very little energy for the relationship with my husband, and I was well aware that I was not very pleasant to be around at that time. For both of us it was a question of just trying to get through each day. We did manage to go out one evening a week for a movie or dinner. I thought to save our marriage we had to at least do that. We also went to a marriage counselor, but this turned out to be a waste of time, as the therapist had no idea what it meant to raise a child with autism. She didn't seem able to relate to the stresses that were rocking our marriage. I ended up feeling misunderstood and resentful and never went to a marriage counselor again.

The Way Out of the Darkness

One day, after about a year of this daily struggle with no significant improvement, I got an unexpected phone call. I will never forget this day because it would change our lives forever. It was an old friend from Boston I had met when I first started RDI. She visited us once with her husband and her two children. One of her sons had autism. Back then I was amazed how well she implemented RDI in her life. She was an unbelievably dedicated mother. Now she called me and told me that she had been reading some of my bio-medical questions on the Internet. She knew of a woman in Maine who maybe could help me and she recommended a web site and a book written by that mysterious woman. I will be always thankful for this phone call because it was the beginning of the long journey back to health and wellbeing for Jimmy. The woman's name was Amy Yasko.

Chapter 6

On the Way to Recovery

Biomedical Intervention with the Amy Yasko Protocol

Biomedical Approaches and the Critics

When most people think of finding "cures" for various health conditions they generally think of some pharmaceutical treatment, or if it were a more clear-cut physical malady then surgical intervention would be considered. Rarely does it occur to them that adjusting diet and taking supplements might favorably influence the condition. Certainly I belonged to this school of thought and it initially never crossed my mind that my son's condition could be improved through taking vitamins and supplements. It was only after my ceaseless digging on the Internet that a small window in my mind was opened to this as a possibility.

Many parents of autistic children will know what I mean when I say that after several interventions have been tried without any success, a desperation takes hold to find something, anything, no matter how far out of the ordinary it might seem.

It is unfortunately true that of the many interventions for autism available, only very few have been shown to be successful in clinical research trials. When I talk about supplements and diets I usually get a lot of criticism. People argue that there is no scientific evidence that vitamins and diets have any effect on autism. The New York Times recently reported that there was no effect on different health conditions when certain vitamins were taken, and that some vitamins made certain health conditions worse. It seems that the jury is still out on the question of vitamin efficacy, but of course there has been fascinating research from the Nobel Prize winner Linus Pauling on the wide-ranging benefits of Vitamin C. Health food stores do brisk business with people clearly convinced that supplements are improving their health. I do feel strongly that there have not been nearly enough studies done on vitamins and health, and I would love to see more investigation into the connection between autism and diets or supplementation.

I am one of those people who started giving her child vitamins. I saw therapists; a psychologist and I tried to see a child psychiatrist. None of those professionals and certainly no scientists were able to help my child get better. I was either informed that nothing was wrong with Jimmy, or there was nothing that could be done about his autism. On the whole, the message from therapists and "experts" was that Jimmy might improve a little but that I more or less had to accept the way he was. It was a bleak outlook and a rather unhelpful "wall" that was placed in front of us.

A Very Different Message from some Parents

However, there was a very different message from some parents of autistic children who had seen their children dramatically improve or even recover when they used biomedical interventions. Because parents were conscious of the risks of certain vitamins many of them looked for professionals with a background in both the biomedical field and nutrition. Reading such reports fuelled my determination to continue searching, and my efforts bore fruit when I found the Amy Yasko protocol, which together with RDI helped my son to full recovery.

This protocol differs greatly from other biomedical approaches in that it uses nutrigenics -- the study of the relationship between the genes and nutrition. She provides an individualized supplemental program based on genetics with the goal of meeting nutritional needs and supporting detoxification of viruses and metals.

Yasko is highly specialized in nutrition and biomedical approaches. She agrees more research needs to be done in this field but she also is aware of the urgent need of parents to find help for their autistic children. When I first heard about her I wrote e-mails to all the biomedical support groups I had found on line to find out if any parents had tried it, and if they had, what they thought about it. The responses were very positive and encouraging, as there was clearly a lot of respect for Amy Yasko, and those that had tried her protocol recommended it.

I had never come across any biomedical approach that seemed to have had as much success as that protocol.

It was highly encouraging that parents of even severely autistic children had had some success with the Yasko protocol when all other treatments had failed. Naturally there were also criticisms. Many parents could not afford the relatively high costs of the supplements and ongoing testing. Other parents complained about the behaviors caused by detoxification and some believed that children should be able to get their nutrition from food alone.

Coming to Grips with the Amy Yasko Protocol

My friend who had been using the protocol on her son and had fully researched it, advised me to thoroughly read Amy Yasko's book and to learn as much as I could. I found the protocol hard to understand and her website was full of terms I had never heard of. Nonetheless I ploughed on and read amazing stories of progress. Fortunately there was a tremendously helpful online discussion forum where I could ask any question I wanted, and this helped greatly in coming to grips with what this protocol was all about.

AMY YASKO BELIEVES THERE IS NO SINGLE CAUSE OF AUTISM

Amy Yasko believes there is no single cause of autism, but that environmental issues and the genetic make-up of the child might play a significant role in autism. Some children are not able to properly detoxify metals, viruses and bacteria because of their genetics and therefore the child needs to be tested for specific genetic mutations, which might be involved in detoxification and methylation. Methylation is a biochemical pathway that is involved in detoxification, immune function, maintaining DNA, energy production, mood balancing and controlling inflammation.

According to its individual mutations the child needs to take supplements in order to support organs and methylation cycles. Usually people start the Yasko protocol by testing the child for genetic mutations. The supplementation requires three steps: organ support, methylation support, and remyelination of the nerves.

During that process Yasko requires that regular metal excretion testing be done. She also emphasizes the importance of regular mineral and amino acid testing. This way Yasko can determine where the child is in the detoxification process, enabling her to make suggestions for further supplementation.

In the first step we started with testing Jimmy for any imbalances in his methylation to determine which supplements he needed for his own profile. Due to our tight financial situation, I kept testing to a minimum and only gave the absolutely necessary supplements to support organs and the balance of the neurotransmitters GABA and glutamate. I added supplements to support aluminum excretion, as well as vitamins that support a healthy digestive system. I started the supplements one at a time at a very low dose in case they triggered heavy detoxification, which apparently could bring on a lot of challenging behaviors.

Yasko makes it clear that this treatment is a marathon rather than a sprint, and indeed we stayed on this step for an entire year. I have to admit that in spite of reading all the positive reports I still had somewhat low expectations. I had tried so many treatments with only minor lasting success, and couldn't banish the thought that this would be just like the others, but I kept at it because you never really know until you have tried something!

When we came to the second step, I added the new supplements really slowly and at very low doses. These supported methylation and targeted chronic bacterial as well as viral issues. Yasko believes that is quite common for autistic individuals to have several bacterial issues such as streptococcal infections as well as multiple viral infections. Viruses such as herpes may exacerbate heavy metal retention in the body. Bacterial loads may also make it harder for the body to excrete toxic metals, thus possibly weakening the immune system. Bacteria are usually treated with antibiotics and viruses are fought with aggressive medications. Yasko believes that those treatments might not be sufficient, and we need to start paying attention to toxic metal excretion, bacterial issues, viral issues and genetics. When I really went into the objectives of this treatment I found it both intriguing and highly interesting.

After two years on the Yasko protocol we finally moved on to step 3: nerve growth and myelination, which is necessary for proper nerve function. Yasko believes that nerves of certain autistic people have been demyelinated from viruses, metals and certain other harmful substances. During this phase we also experienced some regressions with more crying when tired and very noticeable hyperactivity in the evenings.

The reader will have noted that I have not gone into the details of this protocol. Neither have I given a complete overview. There is a very good reason for this. As each child is very different, any parents interested in using this protocol for their child would have to thoroughly educate themselves about the program. It is also a very comprehensive treatment that is changing constantly as new discoveries in the autism field come to light. Amy Yasko is always looking for answers for desperate parents and her website, http://www.holistichealth.com provides help and information on the latest discoveries and advances.

Our Results with the Yasko Protocol

Jimmy's undermining anxiety began to noticeably decrease on this protocol. He seemed calmer and stopped clinging to me all the time. This was a kind of liberation for me -- to be free to move around by myself at last felt amazing. Jimmy even started to play with his neighborhood friend again, and I found myself standing at the fence smiling broadly as they rode their bikes. Normal life was returning to us! When we went to the zoo, Jimmy took a great interest in the animals whereas before he had simply stared blankly at them with no reaction whatsoever! It did seem that he was really coming back to life again.

There were so many improvements at this time but perhaps the most completely transformative milestone on the Yasko protocol was that Jimmy actually started communicating instead of just asking the same questions over and over. This new ability made him seem so much less autistic. I had always used declarative language with him when we were doing RDI but this had no improving effect until we started the Yasko protocol. This combination seemed to be the trigger for the great leap forward which changed so much in our lives. He even started showing us affection for the first time.

There also was a radical improvement in his fine motor skills. For example, suddenly he was able to hold his pen properly when drawing. I had practiced this with him for a long time without any success at all and had subsequently given it up but now he just started holding his pen perfectly. Equally satisfying was the morning when he just got up and dressed himself. Fully dressed he stood in front of me smiling. I could scarcely believe my eyes as we had also practiced this repeatedly, but it had always ended with tears and frustration.

In general Jimmy became much healthier. His teeth turned white again and the rings under his eyes disappeared. He complained a lot less about stomachaches, and no longer had a bloated belly. Interestingly, he also started to get the normal childhood sicknesses just like other kids. Previously he wouldn't get sick but constantly had a runny nose or a cough, and he would cry a lot. Now he started getting fevers, and instead of crying he would just sleep all day. In other words he had become just like my friend's typical children when they were sick. My friends had told me that their children were easier to handle when they were sick. I never understood what that meant until this new development. His body was now working normally and so was his mind.

The Yasko Protocol accelerated progress with RDI

Being on the protocol made it easier for Jimmy to master new objectives in RDI. He seemed to be moving forward without even much practice. As we had been stuck for a quite a while this was a great relief. We practiced telling jokes to each other. Jimmy got it very quickly and I was able to tell the knock, knock joke in many variations. He even came up with his own jokes. That my son was sitting in front of me and telling me a joke was simply unbelievable. Not only was he was now a lot more present and alert, but he seemed to be starting to enjoy life. When he got hurt or upset he could now regulate himself, and would calm down quickly instead of crying for long periods. In fact when he was hurt he would just snuggle against me instead of pushing me away. How I had longed for this day!

When I showed my RDI consultant the new videos I had taken, she was amazed by the transformation. She also noticed that Jimmy was now progressing in RDI a lot faster, and she thought that soon he would no longer need RDI. She confessed that she had not believed that biomedical interventions could make a difference, but after observing all this she started thinking that supplements could be a critical factor for some autistic children. It felt immensely reassuring to be supported in my biomedical approach. This was especially important because regressions did happen from time to time, and then I often had to go slower with RDI.

Getting Beyond Food Sensitivities and A Restricted Diet

Under the Yasko Protocol even the food sensitivities that had plagued Jimmy for so long finally started to improve greatly. On a camping trip Jimmy, by mistake, ate a whole fork full of his friend's wheat pasta and, amazingly, had no reaction. What a break-through. It had been very difficult to justify such a strict diet to critical family and friends and now I could even give Jimmy small amounts of gluten. It was liberating to no longer have to constantly watch him like a hawk to protect him from gluten, though I still kept it to a minimum in his diet. Birthday cake at his friend's birthday parties was no longer off-limits, and he could finally have the same treat as his friends. Even dairy became possible though I kept it out of his food as much as I could, along with artificial colors, flavors and preservatives.

What relief to have finally got beyond the interminable frozen fish sticks, and to be able to add some fruit and vegetables. My husband always fervently wished Jimmy could just sit down with us and eat whatever we were eating. This dream came true, and now we have one meal for the whole family. I still have to sometimes encourage Jimmy to eat veggies by giving him a treat at the end, but I don't think this is very different from how parents of typical kids act.

Finally Off to School

The protocol sped up the progress in relationship skills to the extent that after all those years my little boy was actually able to go off to school. Being healthier definitely helped him deal better with the more complex social situations in groups of peers. He was able to pay better attention to what was going on in the classroom, and being less tired meant he could deal much better with the long, demanding school day. I never thought that would happen so it really did feel like a miracle. Towards the end of the protocol he could do his schoolwork independently, figure things out on his own and make his own friends.

Regressions Are Bound to Happen

When I started the Yasko protocol with Jimmy I noticed that when I gave him certain supplements he would be up for hours at night tossing and turning. Some days he was very rigid and cried easily. Other days he just seemed have forgotten how to play with other children, but I knew by then that those regressions were to be expected and no cause for concern. Occasionally Jimmy would get in a mood where he refused to do every activity I offered, even the ones he liked.

Although his sensitivity to touch and noises improved, and I no longer had to brush him with a plastic brush, occasionally his sensitivity to touch returned for a while, but was never as severe as before the protocol. He remained sensitive to high-pitched noises such as screaming kids at the play space, and it took a longer time and further RDI work before Jimmy was comfortable in larger groups.

Facing Skepticism

I still face skepticism from my scientifically minded husband about the cause of Jimmy's progress. He thinks there is no proof that the Yasko protocol had anything to do with it. I will have to keep an open mind but I do sincerely hope there will be more research on the effects of this protocol on autism. Like many other parents I did not have time to wait for this. My son is doing wonderfully well today, and in my mind there is no doubt that Yasko's approach was a key factor in his recovery from autism.

The Things that Helped Me Through

When I look back, it is clear to me that one of the most vital elements that carried me through this whole process was having access to the discussion group on the Yasko website. Being able to ask questions and educate myself by staying in contact with other people who were doing the same protocol was incredibly helpful. When new supplements did bring on regressions the group, the information I received from Amy Yasko gave me great comfort that they would pass.

I do believe that connecting with other parents was one of the most helpful things I did.

Their experience has been priceless, and no professional advice could have replaced that. Probably none of these marvelous things would have happened without the Internet! Let me sing a short hymn of praise! The Internet was where I met so many people, had so much support and found ways to open my mind and grow. I was lucky that my challenging times coincided with this democratization of information and experience.

In Conclusion

Finally it must be said that not all the parents who tried this protocol saw their children progress. No one therapy will help all autistic children in the same way. Though it can be very hard, you have to keep on searching for the best approach for your child. I am also aware that not every family will be able to afford the Amy Yasko protocol. In this case, there are simple things parents can do to make their children healthier. Many believe that a beneficial effect will come from taking a multivitamin and probiotics, as well as cutting out sugar, artificial colorings and flavors. Indeed many hyperactive children have reverted to "normal" behavior on having artificial colorings, flavors and sugar eliminated from their diet. As many autistic children are picky eaters, there will often be great resistance to change, making implementing a healthy diet very challenging. If this is the case, be very patient and start with minimal changes in a child's diet. Although it may take many years to achieve any significant change toward a healthier and more balanced diet, it is definitely worth persevering in this area.

Chapter Seven

THE CHALLENGE OF MAKING FRIENDS

From Dyads and Groups to School

Imagine a childhood without a best friend, or worse, without any friends. No play dates, sleepovers or birthday parties. You are trying hard to fit in, but you just don't understand other people's actions and feelings. You are trying very hard to play with the other children, but you are failing miserably. A significant percentage of children with autism never succeed in making a true friend.

When left feeling isolated and rejected, low self-esteem is not far behind, and this in turn often leads to anxiety, frustration and behavioral problems. Many of these children isolate themselves and engage in repetitive activities to give them some feeling of security in what seems to them to be a chaotic and scary world. Typically they might spend hours rolling a toy car back and forth or line up their toys instead of actually playing with them. They might spend hours just opening and closing doors, ignoring everyone around them. The social world can seem so overwhelming for them that they often avoid social encounters wherever possible.

As mentioned earlier, one of the main goals in RDI is the ability to develop true friendship with another human being. RDI supporters do not believe that the child can learn friendship skills by just being with other children in a classroom, and therefore special strategies have to be employed to break down the barriers that surround the isolated child.

After mastering being in a guided relationship with a trusted adult, the child is then ready to work with one other child to establish a "partnership". This is called a dyad. For a dyad to work optimally both children should have similar relationship skills and motivations. Otherwise the more skilled child might do all the relationship work. Later on, another child can be added so that the child also learns how to be confident in a group.

A dyad is different from a play date in that the guiding adult in a dyad creates situations where both children are required to work together. The goal is for them to stay together and be equal partners in this task. Both children would start to work at stage one in RDI, and work their way up to higher stages. This all made sense to me.

The Steps Towards Building Social Connections

1. Building up a trusting relationship between parent and child
2. Developing a "dyad" or partnership with another child
3. Adding in a third child
4. Trying appropriate supervised group activities

Making a Dyad Work

Our consultant didn't have a child at Jimmy's level of functioning, and I had no idea how to find an appropriate partner. When no one responded to the notice I posted, I turned to our own neighborhood where I already had connections to neighbors with children of Jimmy's age. I had to find parents who not only trusted us but would also be interested in their child getting practice in relationship skills. Working in my favor was the reality that all mothers feel the need of a break and my working with their child would provide that. Luckily I found a neighbor whose son had known us for over a year. The other mother left us alone, which was a definite advantage as it made it easier for the dyad partner to become my apprentice and to accept me as a guide. It turned out that this child was not the ideal dyad partner as he was clearly ahead of Jimmy in his relationship skills, but he was all that I had to work with at that time so we went ahead with it.

Leading a dyad required much preparation and thought. It was important that both boys kept their attention on each other instead of me. My job was to set up the activity and make sure they had enough time to communicate with each other about how to solve the task. That they themselves figure out how to work together is key. For example, with a beanbag activity that worked well, the task was that the boys should jump together into the beanbags. At the beginning one boy was jumping ahead of the other, and instead of telling them to stay together I would spotlight where they had gone wrong by saying, "Oops you were not together." When this still didn't work, I would jump with them holding hands all together, and if still it wasn't right I would always state that we were not quite together. Gradually they would be able to jump by themselves, making sure they stayed together.

As the boys got better working with each other, I took them to a play space, where for the first time I could just sit on the bench and watch. I was amazed how fast Jimmy's partner moved from one activity to another. Jimmy had no trouble with the fast transitions, and he was now using all the skills we had practiced over the years. They climbed, jumped, played with the trains and chased each other, being constantly in motion and searching for new exciting play. There was Jimmy laughing and playing, having the best time, not with me, but with his own friend.

Our move to the West Coast meant finding a new dyad partner for Jimmy. We were very lucky that our new neighbor had a neurotypical son of around Jimmy's age and needed childcare. The boys liked each other instantly and so I scheduled a dyad for once a week. One of their favorite activities was finding objects they were hiding from each other. I would set up three beanbags, and one boy was hiding a treasure under one of them and would point with his eyes to where the item was hidden. The other boy had to read these signs to find the treasure. Over time they created more complicated treasure hunts, hiding items in the house or the garden. Soon the boys grew fond of each other, and I remember getting woken up often in the morning by the doorbell ringing and both boys begging, "Can we play?"

When they seemed ready, I started taking them into many different environments: playgrounds, fast food restaurants, indoor play spaces and stores. It was important to me that Jimmy learned how to be in a relationship in more complicated environments. For example, practicing doing several tasks at once was possible in a grocery store. He had to be able to watch his friend, stay together with him, but at the same time pick out an item and manage not to run into other customers. At first he still appeared very anxious and overwhelmed in those crowded spaces and would start clinging to me. It was clear where his challenges lay, and this showed me we had a long way to go.

Once Jimmy could interact well with one child, I had to find a way to include more children. One good way of doing this was to bring fun toys with me when we went to the playground or café. Children would flock around us, and this gave Jimmy practice playing in groups. Back then I still had to scaffold all the play between him and the other children, and I have to admit that this was a lot of work.

It still sometimes happened that Jimmy would refuse to go to the coffee house or the playground, and I would have to stand firm and take him anyway. Once he protested and demanded to know why we had to do this every day, and then started crying so loudly that everybody in the coffee house was staring at us. Heaven only knows what they were thinking but it probably wasn't anything positive about me! I retreated in embarrassment, and decided on this occasion there was nothing for it but to take him home. However I resolved to try again the very next day. Most of the time, once he was involved in the play, he would forget that he hadn't wanted to go. Although those play opportunities were worthwhile, there was the problem that the children came irregularly leading me to want to set up a more consistent group.

I often took him to a child friendly, fast food restaurant in our neighborhood. I noticed that the workers brought their children every afternoon to play there. This was a consistent group of children Jimmy could play with! As always, I had plenty of fun learning materials on hand and those children were only too happy to join in. Here was Jimmy learning in a group situation just as he would be doing at school, with the added bonus that he might make a group of new friends.

One fun project I did with those children in the winter was to make snowmen out of different materials such as paper, buttons and beads. They all went together, and decorated the restaurant with their creations. Jimmy made his own snowman and showed it proudly to all the other children. They all had big smiles when the customers admired their artwork. It was the perfect play environment for Jimmy, and I worked with him and those children for many months! I would justify being there by always having a coffee in front of me, and naturally the working parents were delighted to see their children being part of these projects.

Jimmy kept on making great progress and one day I decided to film him and his dyad partner during natural play without me taking part in any way. My consultant had never seen him in "natural" unstructured play with another child, and surprised me completely by declaring that Jimmy would not need RDI any more. I was ecstatic! He had accomplished so much. After that life became a lot more normal.

Enrolling in classes

I was confident that Jimmy was now ready to join some children's sports class. It would still have to be highly structured at the beginning, and it was best to start with a small group. Our first attempt was a karate class, which turned out to be a failure, as Jimmy had a hard time understanding the directions and names of the karate movements. The teacher put constant demands on the kids, and there was little time to think. It made me aware that even though we had come so far; Jimmy was still very different from other children.

I later tried him in a gymnastics class but that was also a disaster. It was a noisy boys-only class, and the exercises were too advanced for him. Not willing to give up, I then put him in a girls' gymnastic class with a female teacher. She made the exercises really fun, and made sure every child stayed confident. Jimmy loved her instantly. This beginner class was perfect for him as the teacher set up "rounds of activities". For example, first the kids would jump on the trampoline, then do five rolls and then climb on the bars and so on. Each child had to watch for his or her turn and when they had mastered the activities the teacher added variations. This was very similar to RDI. Jimmy managed all the activities and also watched the others so that he would not bump into anybody.

Soon I asked the other mothers to watch Jimmy, as I wanted to leave the class to see if he could manage without me being there. At first I just left for five minutes but soon I was able to leave for thirty minutes. It turned out that Jimmy had not missed me at all! This marked real progress, and he continued in this class until he started school at the age of five.

After the successful gymnastic class I tried him in a basketball class. Unfortunately there was such a high turnover of teachers and students that it became much too chaotic for Jimmy. Often the children were unruly, and would run around screaming wildly which made him very anxious. I always stayed close by, and gave him frequent breaks if he got too overwhelmed. In the end I felt that most of those classes did contribute to Jimmy's later success in school, even though there was little chance of any friendships developing there.

Some Home Schooling

With Jimmy's fifth birthday in sight it was time to think about his schooling. I knew that academically he was ready for school, but his social skills still lagged behind. The best option seemed to be to home school him, so I started teaching him reading, phonics, basic math and handwriting. Learning became fun for him when I used a wonderful music program called callirobics. It teaches simple handwriting exercises with music to improve eye-hand coordination, fine motor skills and concentration. There were fun songs to help with practicing simple shapes, letters and numbers. I kept the sessions very short, and made sure there were plenty of playtimes during the day. Jimmy was a fast learner, and made good progress in reading math and writing.

Finding the Ideal School

Other social opportunities developed naturally, such as when I often picked up Jimmy's dyad partner from school, and he ended up playing with the children there. The school was small, and the playground environment was so positive and non-threatening that Jimmy loved going there. I was delighted to see him getting this spontaneous unstructured playing in groups practice. One day when Jimmy was almost five, I was chatting with the principal there, and she told me she thought Jimmy would fit in well at that small school.

I was thrilled about this possibility but realized it might be hard to convince my husband to put our son in a private school, as we lived in an area with supposedly good public schools. Before broaching this I decided to have a closer look at our local public school, and went to check it out. I noticed immediately the big class sizes, and the uninspiring outdoor facilities. The children were outside on the asphalt in the burning summer heat with no trees for protection at break time. The school was fenced all around with big signs declaring unauthorized persons were forbidden to enter school property. The parents had to wait outside the fence for their kids. The school appeared more like a prison than a school to me. The elementary school was big and impersonal with a huge high school next door.

The day I picked up the enrollment papers teachers kept reminding me that I had no authorization to be in the school grounds. I couldn't quite see how I could get the enrollment papers without entering the school grounds. When I finally found the enrollment office, the administration staff was rude and unfriendly, and I just could not picture Jimmy in this environment. There was no comparison with that private school with its small class sizes, beautiful tree-filled yard, rock climbing walls and natural play structures.

Perhaps the deciding factor was that Jimmy had already made friends there. After I talked to my husband, he was also convinced that it would be better for a child like Jimmy to be in a smaller school with a higher teacher to pupil ratio. Somehow we would find a way to pay for it. Jimmy would be enrolled in first grade and would be in a class with twelve other children and mostly two teachers in the classroom. He would be able to work independently at the level of his skills, whatever grade he was in.

The school made a very peaceful and organized impression on me. It had only three classrooms combining different age groups, and there would be plenty of time to play with peers in different environments, such as on hikes, in the playground, in the swimming pool or on excursions.

When I made the appointment for Jimmy to be evaluated, he had to go with the principal all by himself so that she could test him. I was not only really nervous about whether Jimmy would be all right without me, but also about how he would do with the tasks he would be asked to perform. About twenty minutes later both of them came back smiling. He had done it; he had separated from me with a woman he barely knew.

After that Jimmy went off to play with the other kids. There was no doubt at all that this would be a good school for him. He would be happy here. The test had been pretty challenging. He had to write some words, read a list of words and write some numbers. All the work I had done with Jimmy came together on this one day. I could not believe it: my son was going to school, to a regular school without any aid. This was a pure miracle after all we had been through.

Three weeks later Jimmy had his first day in school, and he did just fine. Funnily enough, I was the one who was a mess. I thought I wouldn't make it through the day. I was expecting a call from the teacher to tell me Jimmy was crying, but in fact nothing like that ever happened. The teacher knew about Jimmy's history and my concerns but I didn't get the impression that she took me seriously. This was really good news, as she thought Jimmy was a great kid with nothing "wrong" with him at all. Jimmy did so well with the other children partly because there were mostly girls in the class, and they usually seemed a little calmer than the boys. Six months later when five more boys entered the class, the dynamics changed, and often the somewhat wild boys seemed to overwhelm Jimmy. He reacted by spending more time playing by himself, or watching the other kids. Luckily, in this school I could always observe the playtime, so I noticed the change in him right away.

To overcome this difficulty, I brought lots of games that he could play together with the boys. Those games provided some structure in the play, which he still needed. This made a big difference, and after a few weeks he started playing very actively with all the kids.

It was definitely a good learning experience for him. The teacher fosters a lot of independence and lets the pupils have their unstructured free times, thus allowing them to take responsibly for themselves. I considered this to be vital for Jimmy's development, and was very pleased with this set-up.

Enabling Jimmy to become competent in groups required a tremendous amount of work and time. Playing in a group is very much more dynamic than playing with one child. Many hours of practice were needed. I think his school provides an excellent framework for learning how to play in a group without being intrusive. I had enjoyed home schooling Jimmy, but it was too much effort to keep up his "social" life.

General Thoughts on Setting up a Dyad

- Given that each autistic child has its own individual strengths and obstacles, finding a dyad partner in RDI can be a great challenge. Often families with a potential dyad partner may live too far away to make regular meetings work.
- If a parent's consultant lives close by, parents can ask if their RDI consultant could offer a social group. This can also lower costs.
- Younger typical siblings are often the best dyad partners and can offer plenty of practice every day. Parents can set up dyad–like situations at home, and give their autistic child more and more responsibility in working out the relationship with their siblings. Often the sibling becomes the autistic child's best friend. Older siblings are less ideal since they tend to do more work in the relationship and overcompensate for the challenges the autistic child has. In families with more than two children, parents need to start with a dyad of only one sibling, and after this is mastered, they can add a third child.
- For younger children a quieter playground can offer better possibilities for play. Parents need to be close by and ready to scaffold if necessary, but at the same time giving the child space to figure things out.
- Indoor play spaces, being usually enclosed, can be very good, safe locations, as the child cannot easily run off. Parents should choose the least crowded time so that their child does not get overwhelmed.

General Advice on Schooling Options

I don't believe that large public school classrooms are appropriate places for autistic children to learn social skills. The curriculum is covered, but such an environment might be unable to provide social learning. If parents can't afford a smaller private school or a Special Needs School, they might consider homeschooling and get together with other homeschoolers for "play dates."

Funding

Unfortunately there is very little funding available beyond special needs public education, and parents will mostly have to use their own resources. Engaging in long IEP battles and court cases fighting for aid is seldom a fruitful endeavor. It takes precious time and energy away from the child, and in our straightened economic times those battles seldom lead to success.

Finding a more affordable consultant who offers social groups, and home schooling your child might be the best options parents have. Parents can support each other in home-schooling communities by trading days and sharing each other's responsibilities.

Social life can be very complex. There are the close friends, new friends, older friends, younger friends, groups of friends, and those friends have their own personalities and interests. There are different ever-changing environments where those friendships take place. We might meet friends at our house, or at a friend's house, we might go the park or for a hike. It is a very dynamic process. All this is not easy for a child with autism, and there is no denying that for us it was a long bumpy road to get to the point where our son was comfortable in these various settings. Life is teaching us new things all the time, and we all continue to be challenged in small ways as we meet new friends and keep up relationships with old friends. One thing is certain – our life is now so much richer and more rewarding, as we see our son thriving in a way we could never have expected.

Chapter Eight

RECOVERY

What Does Recovery Mean?

How do we know when a child has recovered? Is it when the child loses the autism diagnosis or when he or she is able to act like neuro-typical youngsters? No longer having the diagnosis doesn't necessarily mean all autistic traits have disappeared. Some parents reported their child remained awkward in social situations even after losing the diagnostic label.

In behavior therapies children learn compensatory strategies to be in a typical developing range, and these may not address the underlying mechanisms. Therefore can you really say that a true recovery has taken place? Skeptics believe a recovered child might have been initially misdiagnosed, and with the autism diagnosis being empirical in nature, there is no way to successfully rebut this view. To complicate matters further, other medical conditions might overlap with symptoms of autism.

There is evidence that the immune system may play a role in autism. Although the focus was previously on the child's immune system in the out-of-favor vaccine-autism link, some scientists have come to believe that infections affecting the mother-to-be during pregnancy can increase the risk of autism in the child. Those findings can be only applied to a subgroup of individuals, and it leads to the question of whether we need to rethink how we define autism.

It seems that just as no one is certain about the complex causes of autism, there is also disagreement about its end point. It may be surprising to hear that recovery is not always a popular term. Some parents of high functioning autistic children ask for more tolerance and understanding instead of a cure. They see autism not as a progressive disorder, but rather as a neurological variation – just part of their particular personality.

A group of people with Asperger's Syndrome (a high functioning form of autism) feels that if we try to get rid of autism we are trying to get rid of them as well. I have seen happy and contented autistic children who presented very little trouble to their parents. They were talking and they were very smart. I can well see how a parent of such a child would be less concerned. Obviously the highly impaired group is more desperate for a cure. In our own case not a day went by where I didn't think Jimmy needed serious help. Our family life was so profoundly affected by his autism, that I spent every minute of my time working on his recovery.

Should the Diagnosis be Kept from the Child?

Another question facing parents of recovered children is whether to disclose the former label to an unaware child, friends or teachers. For example our son was only two years old when he was diagnosed, and now at age five, he has no memory of having autistic symptoms. Parents often decide not to tell out of fear that a former diagnosis could still limit their child's opportunities in life. I decided it was important for Jimmy to know about the autism because there was always a chance that family members or friends might tell him later. Making a secret of the diagnosis might give him the message that having special needs is something "bad." I also told him that he was not autistic any longer and did not give any more details as after all he is very young and it seemed unnecessary.

Why I think of Jimmy as "Recovered"

I think of Jimmy as a recovered child since today he is just a typical boy with many friends and a wide range of hobbies. After all the extreme difficulties we went through it still seems almost incredible to me that he is now so happy and well adjusted. It is fascinating to see how his earlier obsessions have turned into meaningful assets. He used to throw balls randomly in the air and scream for hours if I tried to catch one, but now he loves playing soccer, baseball, basketball and juggling. He used to count all day and stare obsessively at the temperature display in the car, but now he is working at above his grade level in math. This year he is even on the nationwide Kumon honor roll in math. Instead of screaming for hours when another child wanted to play with him, now he can't stop talking about a sleepover at his friend's house. His pleasure in his friends is so strong that sometimes he goes to bed earlier at night, explaining that this way he will have his play date sooner!

Jimmy's behavior can still drive me mad, but now it is caused by more normal impulses such as sneaking over to his friend's house without asking me! Whenever I find myself getting annoyed about something like this, I remind myself that previously he never wanted to go to anybody's house at all. When I see him wrestling with another child I can barely believe that he used to be terrified of any kind of touching.

The Triumph of Succeeding in Relationships

Building friendships with peers is so very difficult for autistic children, and for Jimmy too, having a relationship with another child was one of the most difficult things of all. Given that fact, seeing him these days playing so well in groups and being popular amongst girls and boys of all ages is truly wonderful. He also has a best friend with whom he loves to play and have adventures.

As children get older peer relationships become more important and more complex. RDI has prepared Jimmy well for making real friends, and has enabled him to maintain friendships. I know of very young autistic children who were doing well connecting with others, but later it became too difficult for them to keep up with their peers' social skills. In the more advanced stages of RDI the child gets increasingly challenged in more complex peer situations. For example, Jimmy really wanted to have a play date with a girl at his school. As he likes bowling he said he would like to invite her to go with him. I asked him what he would do if she said she didn't want to do this. He said, "Oh, then we can do something we both like." He clearly understands that in order to have a friendship both of them have to have a good time.

Mastering School

It is very rare for an autistic child to be able to attend a regular school with no special help and to flourish in that environment. Our decision to put Jimmy in the very small private school has been clearly the right decision, since he has progressed so well both academically and socially there. It was very helpful that the pupils in Jimmy's school work in study groups switching roles between the apprentice and the master. This approach was very effective with Jimmy, as it was similar to how he had been used to working in RDI. Given that autistic children so often have very poor reading comprehension, it was gratifying to see that this school's enlightened methods even managed to bring Jimmy's comprehension skills up to par with those of his classmates.

He also became highly motivated to enjoy the content of the story rather than just reading the phonics without meaning as he used to. He started telling me the plots of stories they were reading, and would comment on how funny or silly some of the actions of the characters were. His favorite story right now is about a girl who found a crystal rock in her backyard. Her dad taught her all about rocks and crystals, and at the end she put her special rock next to her bed before she went to sleep. Jimmy did the same thing with his favorite rock after we read the story. Reading comprehension opened up a whole new world for him. It also sets the foundation for his future education.

Relating to the Community at Large

Not only has Jimmy mastered building relationships in school but also I have encouraged him to be active in the wider community. Many people, for a variety of reasons, fail to connect with their neighborhoods, and it is particularly difficult for families with autistic children. In spite of our busy schedules we make a point of working hard to get to know other parents and neighbors. I invite them over for a BBQ, we bake cakes for them, or we play games together.

In our neighborhood the people know each other and give each other support. We see them when we ride our bikes on the streets or when we go to the local Farmers' Market. Our kids bake, bike, or play ball together. With his Boy Scout friends he collected food for the homeless in our neighborhood and sang in a local retirement home. This social involvement brings home to us just how far he has come. He clearly got something out of all this and in no way resisted doing these things.

The Power of Relating to the Natural World

It was very important to me that Jimmy was able to develop a relationship with nature. I see this relationship as a spiritual connection. It allows children to see that all life is connected, and that they are part of the earth. Although Jimmy used to hate the water, wind and the sun, spending time outdoors has become a major part of our lives. Finally I can share my passion for the outdoors with my whole family. Today I can't describe the happiness I feel when Jimmy and I go on a hike, build a fort or climb a tree. It's magical to see the huge smile on his face when he is bending down to smell the flowers, or when he is catching beetles or jumping over the waves in the ocean.

At those moments he seems so alive and in tune with where he is. Jimmy often invites his friends on our outdoor excursions, where they spend happy hours in the woods collecting acorns, catching tadpoles and frogs, climbing rocks and trees, or playing in the water. Sometimes I bring ropes to build tree swings. We regularly go on camping trips with friends, renting a cabin in the mountains or on a lake. We have even managed to bring the outdoors into our everyday life by building a tree house in our yard. Sometimes on hot nights we even sleep up there. Over time we all became interested in birding and this has developed into a passion for us. Now that we are freed from that single-minded focus on autism, our whole family has grown closer through these activities, and this has been so healing for us all.

My Own Recovery

The truth is that recovery has not only taken place in my child but also within myself. In the first years of Jimmy's life I was completely unable to be my real self. I was housebound, depressed, and without friends. How badly I needed recovery in those hard years, when even hope deserted me! These days though, I am a completely different person, sharing the same challenges of most mothers, coping with the everyday ups and downs, and enjoying watching my child's growth. I am no longer isolated, and can relax spending time with the other parents and our children.

After five long years of never having a single minute to think about my own needs, I now finally have time for my own interests and hobbies. As a child I loved being out in the woods playing under the trees, or riding horses through the meadows with my best friend. It was this connection with horses and nature that helped me survive those rough times living under Communism. Picking up this thread again after Jimmy's recovery, I found a beautiful quarter mare to lease, and now I love nothing more than being out galloping through the woods.

Having felt shut out from the world for so long makes my new freedom almost heady. I am learning about the wonders of the native plants and animals where we live. This has become such a passion and a pleasure for me that I have recreated a wilderness in my own yard by planting all sorts of native trees and plants. I love sitting in my yard with a cup of coffee when lizards, jays and doves come to visit. Life is once again full of excitement.

When I was all wrapped up with autism, it was the be all and end all of my life. I literally never talked about anything else. This must have been very difficult for other people, and slowly my relationships broke down, until in the end I even stopped talking to my relatives: making my isolation complete. After Jimmy's recovery my depression lifted and I came back to life. It was so rewarding to reconnect with my extended family again and a great joy to go off on hikes with my mother-in-law when she visited. I had really missed this. When I finally knew Jimmy was going to be alright and that he would have friends and enjoy his life, the entire fear and autism fixation just fell away from me. No longer did I have to walk on eggshells: confidence and a feeling of new possibilities opened up before me.

During the long years of struggling with Jimmy's autism, very many times I came up against a wall, questioned my abilities, and even lost faith in myself. Before having Jimmy, I thought I could do anything if I just wanted to do it. I did my high school diploma when I was twenty-nine years old. I completed my Masters degree with honors. Those were things people thought I would never accomplish. But I did it because I thought I could do it. I believed in myself. Life had taught me that if I really want to do something I could do it. Jimmy taught me otherwise. When I had Jimmy it was not about me anymore. It was about another human being I had to put before my own needs. Often I desperately wanted to sleep, but I had to stay up taking care of Jimmy all night. When I was hungry, often I couldn't sit down to eat. If I was lucky I could grab a bite while walking my screaming baby all day long.

In Boston's icy winter with four-foot high snow banks, I had to take Jimmy out to calm him down even though that was the last thing I wanted to do. Knowing that it was not in my power to keep my baby safe and comfortable was torture. I desperately wanted him to be happy like my other friends' babies, but his interminable crying led my friends to start judging me and criticizing me as a mother. I was giving my all, but still I was not successful. I felt like a failure and my spirit was broken.

Having Jimmy was so very different from taking a test in school, learning another language or convincing an employer that I was the right candidate. The truth that things were not in my control depressed me greatly at the time, but now that Jimmy has recovered, I realize that all that pain and suffering has brought clear rewards as well. Just living through this whole experience has significantly changed the way I look at life.

There are some things in life that are not directly in my control and I am now more able to accept that. When I talk to parents who have an autistic child, and tell them that Jimmy has recovered, they usually say, "You are lucky". Yes I am very lucky. I did work very hard with my son but so did many other parents, and their children might not have recovered. It wasn't as if I took a test, scored a 100 % and therefore he recovered. Putting another human being before my own needs was the hardest thing I have ever done.

Jimmy's predicament taught me to be in the moment and worry less about next week or next year. In fact, now I worry much less in general. Sometimes if I plan a day and things turn out completely differently, I find I am quite OK with it. I would have had major trouble with this in the past. These days I am more flexible, calmer and I am able to go with the flow. I cannot have everything I want and I thought I needed, and this too is OK. This is the difference between now and life before Jimmy.

The Recovery Extends to the Wider Family

Jimmy's ordeal has also enabled me to rescue the broken relationship with my parents. Now I have understanding and empathy for them and we finally have the relationship I always wanted. I can call them up any time and discuss everything with them. We both are open now. All the resentment is gone. They had a tough job raising four children in a communist county with very few resources. I have the deepest respect for them. They both sacrificed their needs to feed their children and keep them safe. We are not that different.

Jimmy forced me to grow up and deal with my parents as an adult. For far too long I was stuck in being their child, blaming them for the education they had not given me, or often doing things just to please them instead of making my own decisions.

Having this child made me learn to think for myself. Certainly nobody else had any clear ideas or solutions how to help my child so I was forced to take responsibility, and finally become an independent person. Taking responsibility for myself also enables me to be more assertive in life. I do not have to blame other people anymore if things go wrong. Our family life suffered greatly during the years of our constant struggle with autism. It would be no exaggeration to say that we became a dysfunctional family. We couldn't go anywhere: we could not leave the house with our son or even invite friends and family, as visits were a disaster.

With the recovery, our social life has become normal and all the more enjoyable after years of social isolation. Now every year we visit my husband's family in Colorado. Jimmy so enjoys being with his grandmother; he loves making birdhouses with his uncle and clay pots with his aunt. In Germany his grandfather's dream came true, when he was able to take his first train ride with his grandson. Now everybody in the family enjoys being with Jimmy.

The High Importance of Spending Quality Time as a Family

Today I treasure our life as a family, and I think a lot about how we spend our time. Many middle class Americans' lives are so pressured that parents resort to feeding their kids fast food, and rarely sit down to dinner as a family. Driving children to organized sports and activities can eat into precious family time. As we haven't involved our son in organized sports, we have more time to do things together. We have made the conscious choice of trying to always have our meals together. This is such important quality time: a time for sharing and bonding, and for building closer relationships. Doing this regularly, gives a child a feeling of stability and security.

In today's world even very young children spend a great deal of time with electronics. Clearly children need to be acquainted with computers, but we've always tried to keep electronic games to a minimum, and chosen more life enhancing family activities such as playing board games, going on bike rides, or just being together. I am especially happy about the relationship I see now between Jimmy and his father. My husband's work responsibilities were very great, and I was Jimmy's primary caretaker during those difficult years. He is an engineer and I often faced resistance from him when I was trying scientifically unproven treatments. But now when I see them enjoying their special time throwing a football or making banana bread, I am so glad I persevered. When Jimmy was so sick and miserable, it was impossible for them to do anything together.

Jimmy's successful social interaction has its roots firmly in RDI. Of all the treatments that were part of the recovery mosaic, RDI proved to be crucial in teaching Jimmy about relationships. Now that he has mastered all the RDI objectives, he has gone on to become a great problem solver. Even today I see that RDI is still a useful tool in teaching him to be successful. Sometimes things like gardening or woodworking can be too hard, so I use my RDI toolkit to make the task easier. It is always well worth putting in the extra effort. Now we have lots of fun together, and we are truly "mother and son" at last.

There is No "Right Way" of Treating Autism

This general truth stands out after my five years of researching autism, and working with my own child. After the diagnosis there was no road map to guide us. It was very difficult indeed to know where to start and which therapies to choose.

There are an overwhelming number of treatments available: RDI, Floor time, ABA, Teach, Son Rise Program, the gluten and dairy free diet, homeopathy, auditory listening, detox programs, biological ecology diet, therapeutic horse back riding, occupational therapy, speech-therapy and many more. Although it often might feel very daunting, the reality is that parents may need to try a lot of therapies in order to find what helps their particular child. It might be only one therapy, or a combination of therapies. Parents also need to be aware of side effects or dangers in certain biomedical therapies like chelating. It is left to the parents to navigate this maze of possible therapies and decide which route to follow. This can be very time-consuming on top of having to take care of an autistic child. I discovered that most of the parents who successfully treated their children, used a combination of a behavioral therapy and a biomedical therapy. I have also heard reports from parents who used ABA as the only treatment, and had great success with it. Again, each child is different. Parents need to persevere with one therapy before introducing a second one. It might take months before the child improves, and this trial and error process could well take many years.

I have written Jimmy's recovery story to help parents and children facing autism. I had so many questions when Jimmy was autistic, and I could not find the answers. I lived autism every day for years, working with my son, reading about treatments or surfing on the Internet. This book is a summary of what I learnt about autism, about my family and about myself. I hope that it will give a better understanding of the options and possibilities available to parents of an autistic child.

Difficulties are almost certain along the way. But life is all about change, and nothing stays the same for very long. Our own attitudes determine a great deal. Progress and a new way of being came slowly and surely to us. I hope that the success we found will help parents remain steadfast and never give up trying to find the way that will turn out to be the right way for their own child to improve and possibly recover.

The hero of this story is Jimmy. He did not know how to be in a relationship but the important thing was that he was motivated to persevere. He never gave up and in the end he proved that a child with autism could figure out how to connect with people. I will never forget the early years of Jimmy's life: the pain on his face and his tiny fingers always balled tensely into fists even when he was sleeping. Looking at him just broke my heart. Day after day I would look at him sleeping, hoping he would wake and give me a smile. Instead he would just stare into the light. He did not even register my presence. There was nothing more painful in my life.

Finally now we have the relationship I always wished for. This would have been impossible without his determination to learn to grow and to overcome the many challenges on the way to his recovery. He was the one who took the supplements. He was the one who trusted me to guide him through RDI and he finally trusted himself to reconnect with the world around him. He is the one who says, "I love you mom" before he goes to bed. He is the one who makes my day every day.

THE END

Possible RDI Activities

This is a list of suggestions of activities for working in RDI with your child. All of these I have tried out myself and managed to work with. Of course each child will have different preferences, and probably each parent will end up with a different list. What I have written here is just an indicator of how simple everyday things can be very effective for advancing your child's RDI skills. It's important to understand that the perfect outcome of the task is not the priority: here the crucial focus is on the child and partner working together. The laundry, for example, might not be folded the way you like, but as long as you work on the given objective and the child is an active participant, the RDI goal has been achieved. Parent and child will work on specific objectives given by their consultants. For example, on one occasion the goal might be to throw the laundry into the machine at the same time, while on other occasion the objective might be to take turns at putting the laundry in. As you get into it, it will become clear how endless the opportunities are to do simple everyday RDI activities with your child.

Using Balls:

- throwing, kicking, rolling, bouncing
- variations with different items: throwing oranges, apples, balloons and stuffed animals instead of balls.
- playing basketball: take a laundry basket and toss a ball in there, vary the distances

- crashing balls together
- bowling balls
- bouncing on the ball

Laundry:

- filling up the dryer, filling up the washing machine with clothes
- transferring the laundry from the washer into the dryer
- carrying laundry together
- folding laundry together
- putting laundry into the closet
- when loading the washer and dryer, the parent can mix things up occasionally by, for example, handing the child something that would never be put in the laundry
- sorting laundry together

Outdoor activities:

- ride a tandem bike, scooters, bikes or skateboards together
- take a walk: point out flowers, animals, rocks and other interesting things, walk at different speeds, walk backwards, lead the child by the hand with the child's eyes closed
- go out for a treat: change the route you usually take
- at the beach: run in and out of the water, play in sand, pretend making cookies or something similar out of sand, dig a hole, make sandcastles, chase birds, draw in the sand with your fingers and so on

At the Store:

- push a shopping cart together, take turns pushing the shopping cart, one pushes the card while the other one places items in cart, switch roles, push cart fast, slow, stop and go, spin around
- take a basket instead of a shopping cart, carry the basket together and vary speed, practice stop and go
- referencing which item to buy by nodding and headshaking, smiling and frowning
- coordinate putting items in the shopping basket
- reference which aisles to go to next
- put items on the conveyer belt, the child can hand the items, then reverse roles.
- anticipate: pause before handing the item, bring something funny from home and hand it to child instead of an item from the store
- bring pictures of produce to buy and find them together, put a picture of a family member or pet in between to surprise the child.
- hand shopping items high up or down low, slowly or fast
- coordinate with two shopping carts or two baskets, each having their own

At the Pool:

- swimming on the back together, breaststroke swimming, walking in water together, hopping in water together etc.
- pushing together against the rail, vary the counting for example: one, two, three, two, four, six and so on
- play ball back and forth in the pool

- jump into the pool together, holding hands, or not holding hands, vary the places to jump in from, making big jumps or little jumps
- splash each other
- for a variation use floats and noodles to swim together back and forth

In the Shower:

- vary the water temperature within safe limits
- take turns under the shower
- just wet the feet, arms, or hands
- walk through the shower together
- collect water in a container
- take a long shower, take a short shower and so on

Airplane activities if you travel:

- coloring book, color different parts, use different colors
- take a small drawing board, do hand over drawing with them, take turns drawing and erasing, draw a picture with missing parts that the child needs to fill in, for example, a tree without leaves
- take beads: make a necklace, take it apart, take turns selecting colors and shapes, make the necklace longer and longer
- using stickers: put stickers down at the same time, draw a scene and let the child add stickers to it, take turns putting stickers on each other: nose, forehead, etc

- play dough: make snakes, pizza, choose colors, make big things, little things, make a person, objects or bugs together, use the handover technique if necessary.
- Lego: build a tower together, take it apart, build a structure and let the child copy you step by step

Marble games:

- build a marble labyrinth together
- let marbles run down the track: take turns, alternate number of marbles, colors, if more people participate reference whose turn is next, add pauses so child needs to wait for your turn
- use two cups and pour marbles back and forth
- reference where the marbles are

Pillow and Beanbag activities:

- carry pillows together
- build a pillow mountain
- reference which beanbag to pick up
- run, walk backwards, into a beanbag mountain
- fall into a pillow mountain
- throw, swing the pillows back and forth
- hide under the pillows

  pretend to sleep, wake each other up on the pillow
- make an obstacle course with beanbags
- have a pillow fight

Drum activities:

- ❖ rolling the drum back and forth
- ❖ coordinate drumming: fast and slow, soft and loud, stop and go
- ❖ stick fight with drumsticks
- ❖ drumming on different objects: pots, pens, walls etc

Simple Board games:

- ❖ zingo
- ❖ fishing game
- ❖ cherry game
- ❖ memory games
- ❖ domino
- ❖ go fish
- ❖ candy land

Swinging:

- ❖ swing together on same swing, different swings
- ❖ swing high or low,
- ❖ reference which swing to use
- ❖ catch a ball on the swing
- ❖ sing different songs on the swing
- ❖ pause with each push that the child is anticipating

Baking:

- ❖ pour ingredients together, take turns or hand over

- stir together, take turns or hand over, vary speed
- taste dough together
- shape cookies together, hand prebaked cookies to put on tray
- check if cookies are done
- decorate cookies with sprinkles, M&Ms , nuts or fruit

Cooking:

- mix together, take turns or handover
- cut vegetables together
- put spices on together
- crack eggs together
- pour rice together

Recommended Reading

1) **Autism Asperger's: Solving the Relationship Puzzle** by Steven E Gutstein

Dr. Gutstein is the founder of RDI (Relationship Developmental Intervention). This book describes a six-phase intervention program for teaching people with Autism/Asperger Syndrome to enjoy and participate in meaningful relationships. He explains the social deficits of children with Autism, and provides a step-by-step treatment plan.

2) **The Puzzle of Autism: Putting it all Together: A Guide to Transforming the Treatment of Autism** by Amy Yasko and Gary Gordon

This book presents an overview of the complex and multi-factorial condition of autism. Amy Yasko offers both science and hope for recovery. She shows how to improve the body's detoxification of metals and viruses by nutrigenomics: using nutrition to bypass genetic mutations.

3) **Louder Than Words: A Mother's Journey in Healing Autism** by Jenny McCarthy

This book was written by the celebrity Jenny McCarthy. She describes how behavioral therapy, diet and supplements helped her son recover from autism.

4) **Let Me Hear Your Voice** by Catherine Maurice

An account of how a mother recovered both of her children from autism with ABA (Applied Behavioral Analysis), a behavioral therapy

5) **Unraveling the Mystery of Autism and Pervasive Developmental Disorder** by Karyn Seroussi

Karyn Serousi wrote a practical book about her son's recovery applying and researching extensively the GFCF diet (gluten and casein free diet)

6) **A Real Boy: A True Story of Early Intervention, and Recovery** by Christina Adams

Christina Adams wrote a true story about her son's recovery from autism. She describes different treatment programs such as ABA program, diet, speech, occupational therapy, and medication

7) **Ten Things That Every Child with Autism Wishes You to Know** by Ellen Notbohm

Ellen Notbohm allows the reader to get into the mind of a child with Autism, and shows how he/she perceives the world around them. She tries not to "fix" her son, but rather enter his world and engage him so that he can seek her world out as well

8) **George & Sam: Two boys, One Family, and Autism** by Charlotte Moore

Charlotte Moore writes about the impact of autism on her family and her approach to finding the best ways to help her sons

9) **The Out-of-Sync Child has Fun: Activities for Kids with Sensory Processing Disorder** by Carol Stock Kranowitz

The author describes a fun approach to helping a child with sensory processing challenges

10) **Families of Adults with Autism: Stories and Advice for the Next Generation** by Jane Johnson and Anne Van Rensselaer

A collection of real life stories of autistic adults as told by family members

11) **Finding Ben: A Mother's Journey through the Maze of Asperger's** by Barbara LaSalle

A mother's story about her search to get help and the proper diagnosis for her son

12) **Son Rise: The Miracle Continues** by Neil Kaufman

A father tells the recovery story of his son and describes the creation of the Sun Rise Program

13) **Making Peace with Autism** by Susan Senator

Susan Senator describes her family life and her journey with her autistic son

14) Amalgam Illness, Diagnosis and Treatment: What You Can Do to Get Better, How Your Doctor Can Help by Andrew Hall Cutler

Andrew Cutler discusses diagnosing and treating mercury poisoning from amalgam fillings

15) **Hair Test Interpretation: Finding Hidden Toxicities** by Andrew Hall Cutler

This book tells how to interpret results of hair testing for mercury

16) **The Way I see it: A Personal Look at Autism & Asperger's** by Temple Grandin

Temple Grandin offers practical advice, a great deal of research and her perspective on autism

17) **Thinking in Pictures: My life with Autism** by Temple Grandin

Grandin tells us how thought processes affect the autistic individuals' ability to learn abstract things and socialize with others

18) **Engaging Autism: Using the Floortime Approach to Help Children Relate, Communicate, and Think** by Greenspan and Weider

Greenspan and Weider explain the Floortime approach and offer helpful practical advice to parents who are using this therapy

19) **What Your Doctor May Not Tell You About Children's Vaccinations** by Cave and Mitchell

This book offers parents guidance on making choices about their children's vaccinations

Websites on Autism

http://www.autismspeaks.org/

One of the world's leading science and advocacy organizations for autism

http://www.rdiconnect.com/

How to get started on RDI

http://www.holistichealth.com/

How to get started on the Amy Yasko protocol

http://www.autism.com/

Organization that provides resources for information on autism

Made in the USA
Lexington, KY
05 January 2014